TONICS ❧ OILS ❧ BALMS

The
Simple Guide to
NATURAL
HEALTH

FROM APPLE CIDER VINEGAR TONICS
TO COCONUT OIL BODY BALM,
150+ HOME REMEDIES
FOR HEALTH AND HEALING

MELANIE ST. OURS

ADAMS MEDIA
NEW YORK   LONDON   TORONTO   SYDNEY   NEW DELHI

For Lelia and Dolores

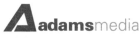

Adams Media
An Imprint of Simon & Schuster, Inc.
57 Littlefield Street
Avon, Massachusetts 02322

First Adams Media hardcover edition August 2018

ADAMS MEDIA and colophon are trademarks of Simon & Schuster.

For information about special discounts for bulk purchases, please contact Simon & Schuster Special Sales at 1-866-506-1949 or business@simonandschuster.com.

The Simon & Schuster Speakers Bureau can bring authors to your live event. For more information or to book an event contact the Simon & Schuster Speakers Bureau at 1-866-248-3049 or visit our website at www.simonspeakers.com.

Interior design by Colleen Cunningham
Interior images © Getty Images/druzhinin-collection, THEPALMER, ivan-96, mashuk

Manufactured in the United States of America

10 9 8 7 6 5 4 3 2 1

Library of Congress Cataloging-in-Publication Data
St. Ours, Melanie, author.
The simple guide to natural health / Melanie St. Ours.
Avon, Massachusetts: Adams Media, 2018.
Includes bibliographical references and index.
LCCN 2018015133 (print) | LCCN 2018017648 (ebook) | ISBN 9781507205655 (hc) | ISBN 9781507205662 (ebook)
Subjects: LCSH: Naturopathy--Popular works. | Alternative medicine--Popular works. | BISAC: HEALTH & FITNESS / Healing. | HEALTH & FITNESS / Alternative Therapies. | HEALTH & FITNESS / Herbal Medications.
Classification: LCC RZ440 (ebook) | LCC RZ440 .S72 2018 (print) | DDC 615.5/35--dc23
LC record available at https://lccn.loc.gov/2018015133

ISBN 978-1-5072-0565-5
ISBN 978-1-5072-0566-2 (ebook)

CONTENTS

Chapter 3

The Healthy Home

43

Chapter 4

Hair, Skin, and Nails

67

⟫ *Chapter 5* ⟪

Immune and Respiratory Systems

97

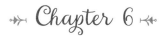

Chapter 6

Digestive Health

123

Chapter 7

Emotional Balance and Mental Health

145

✷ Chapter 8 ✦

Fitness and Flexibility

169

✷ Chapter 9 ✦

Detoxification and Damage Control

191

❧ *Chapter 10* ❧

Women's Health

211

✒ Conclusion ✒

Next Steps and Resources

237

✒ Appendix A ✒

Recommended Reading

243

✒ Appendix B ✒

US/Metric Conversion Chart

246

Index

247

ACKNOWLEDGMENTS

All of the knowledge in this volume has made its way to me through long lineages of tradition spanning at least three continents. To the countless generations of healers and teachers who developed and carried this knowledge for centuries: I remember you with deep gratitude. To Michael and Lesley Tierra, Susan Kramer, Heidi Lindemann and Michael Perry, Christine Lynn, Andrea J. Lee, and all of the teachers and writers who've lit the way for me: thank you. To my clients, students, and community: thank you for being my best teachers of all. Thanks to Julia Jacques, Katie Corcoran Lytle, and the team at Adams Media for making all of this possible. To Ali, Adam, Whitney, and Sara: your help on the manuscript alone would be enough reason to thank you, but you know my love and gratitude don't stop there. Thank you for everything. Special thanks to everyone on the recipe-testing team: Kyoko Bristow, Lisa Mitchell, Carrie James, Kayla Mollet, Anna Keefe, Helen Kinsel, Claire Murphy, Morgan Hodge, Kim Pence, Barbara Elder, Christine Hendrix, Michelle Bobrow, Jessica Grossman, Shannon Mulligan, and Kaitlin Brown. I couldn't have done this without you. Thank you, always, to my family and my ancestors. May my efforts prove worthy of the love you've given and the sacrifices you've made on my behalf.

PREFACE

After six years of clinical practice and many more years of study, my trust in the power of herbal medicine is unshakeable. Herbs aren't miracle cures, but they do happen to be perfectly suited to complement some of the weaknesses of the conventional medical system. Week after week, my clients bring me all manner of physical and emotional woes that conventional medicine has been unwilling or unable to resolve. And month after month, I watch almost all of my clients get better. This high success rate isn't the result of some special talent of mine; it's made possible by the sophisticated understanding of health and disease that constitutes Traditional Chinese Medicine and guides my practice. It's *normal* for our bodies to heal when they're freed from underlying imbalances and supported with a healthy lifestyle. While it takes many years of study to know how (and when *not*) to use herbs to intervene in complex health challenges, the everyday practices that can sustain your health are accessible. This book is all you need to get started.

My sincere wish for you, dear reader, is already within your grasp. I want you to experience the relief, pleasure, and support that herbal medicine has to offer. That's why I've set up this book so that you'll use it, not just read it. Your own direct experience will be your best teacher. Try the remedies. Notice the scents, the subtle shifts in sensation, the way each one makes you feel as you taste it. Trust yourself. If you do, it won't be long before you come to rely on Nature's healing gifts. And once that happens, don't be surprised if in addition to renewed vitality, you find yourself filled with a new sense of gratitude for this beautiful Earth we call home.

INTRODUCTION

Natural medicine works. Our thrifty, creative, no-nonsense ancestors relied on herbal remedies that offer just as many benefits today as ever. *The Simple Guide to Natural Health* teaches a modern version of these time-tested healing traditions and makes it easy to start using medicinal plants, healing foods, and everyday ingredients to help yourself and your loved ones thrive.

The pages of this book contain step-by-step instructions for more than 150 homemade remedies designed to be effective, economical, and easy to prepare. Each chapter focuses on one of your body's major systems and features two kinds of recipes: remedies that relieve common complaints so you can bounce back after an illness, injury, or imbalance; and tonics (including health-supporting foods) you can enjoy regularly to nourish, strengthen, and revitalize your body.

If you've been using natural remedies for years, this book will inspire you with novel ways to use familiar ingredients. The recipes can even serve as templates you can customize to develop personalized formulas for yourself and your loved ones. Or, if you're just getting started, you can rely on this definitive guide to take the guesswork out of the learning process. With this book in hand, you have all the information you need to confidently choose, purchase, and store health-promoting ingredients; understand their benefits; use them safely; and turn them into teas, tinctures, balms, and salves. Before long, you'll be enjoying creations that will transform your home into a sweet-smelling sanctuary; pamper every inch of your skin; sneak powerful antioxidants into your meals; and relieve all kinds of everyday issues, from insomnia to menstrual cramps. Let's get started!

Chapter 1

INTRODUCING THE WORLD OF NATURAL REMEDIES

You belong to Nature. Even amidst the noise and scramble of your busiest days, you are always being held and sustained by the Earth—just like every other creature on this planet. No matter what you eat, how you beautify your skin and hair, or what medicines you reach for when you're suffering, you remain a child of Nature endowed with the right to receive her healing gifts. This book will show you how good it feels to know that you can lean on herbal preparations, healing foods, and natural remedies whenever you need support.

There's a profound feeling of gratitude that comes from realizing just how abundant Nature's gifts really are, yet the day-to-day experience of making and using remedies is entirely practical. There's a reason for each ingredient and a rationale behind every step. Once you understand a few basic principles of herbalism, you'll be ready to shop for ingredients, try your hand at the recipes, and experience the power of natural medicine firsthand. This chapter will give you insight into some of the special properties of herbs, the guiding principles behind natural healing techniques, and how to use natural remedies safely (and when not to use them at all).

Why Use Natural Remedies?

Traditional Chinese Medicine teaches that one way to understand the nature of illness is to picture it as a tree with many branches and a deep root system. The branches represent the various symptoms that cause a sick person to suffer while the root system is the underlying pattern of imbalance that feeds those branches to keep them alive. Cutting off a branch is analogous to treating a symptom; it might bring temporary relief, but it doesn't cure the problem. As long as the root system remains intact, the illness will find new ways to express itself. Unless you uproot the underlying imbalance, it will be only a matter of time before symptoms return.

Think about how you might relieve a tension headache. Popping an ibuprofen might reduce the pain, but if your head hurts because you spent a stressful day hunched over your computer with no time to eat or stretch, that ibuprofen won't get anywhere close to the root of the problem. Unless you change something at work, the pain will keep coming back. It's okay to take something for relief when you need it, but don't stop there! If you take regular stretching breaks, keep a water bottle on your desk so you stay hydrated, and negotiate healthier boundaries with that challenging coworker to reduce your stress, you'll prevent headaches—and be happier. Instead of side effects, natural interventions like these that treat you as a whole person tend to have side *benefits* for your body, mind, spirit, and relationships.

Natural Remedies Encourage Prevention

Even though most people agree that it's ideal to prevent health problems before they start, only a small subset of the population is able to put their knowledge about healthy living into daily practice. It's not always easy to make healthy choices. Living a prevention-focused lifestyle requires you to pay attention to how you feel physically and emotionally, and to prioritize your health despite all kinds of external pressures. Lack of time—and its best friend, stress—often thwarts our plans to live healthier lifestyles. Natural remedies can help—though perhaps not in the way you think.

Since natural remedies can bring quick relief with minimal fuss, they make it easier to respond to your physical and emotional needs without fear that self-care will take too much time away from other important obligations. As you experience the benefits, you'll want to keep taking care of yourself because it *feels* good—not just because you know it's good for you. And the more you learn about health and come to enjoy the pleasurable parts of a naturally healthy lifestyle, the more interested you're likely to be in making other changes that are right for you. You don't have to overhaul your whole life all at once. (Or ever.) A gentle, consistent investment of attention is the key to doing more of what helps you thrive and less of what makes you sick, tired, and stressed. And that's what prevention is all about.

Natural Remedies Awaken Your Senses

Aromatic remedies can revive your senses in a matter of seconds if they've been dulled by stress, mental work, or too much time in front of a screen. A cup of tea or a soothing blend of essential oils can banish mental chatter and bring you into the sensory pleasures of the present moment. Over time, the practice of tuning into your senses pays dividends. The fragrance, flavor, and color of a plant are good clues as to its health benefits, and as you work with natural ingredients, you'll be training your senses to notice these cues. The more you practice, the more you'll find yourself reaching for the herbs, spices, and essential oils that you need without having to consult a book or check the Internet. You'll learn to trust yourself. Sharper senses enhance your enjoyment of life's simplest pleasures. They'll make you a better cook, support your intuition, and maybe even open whole new avenues of enjoyment when you walk through the woods and discover that you recognize subtle sounds and fragrances that you never noticed before.

Natural Remedies Complement Modern Medicine

There's no need to feel conflicted about the choice between natural remedies and over-the-counter or prescription medications. They complement each other perfectly. Modern medicine offers advanced diagnostics, lifesaving emergency treatments, and precise surgical and pharmaceutical interventions for conditions that are impossible to treat on your own. It also includes drug-free approaches to healing, like physical therapy and psychotherapy. Natural remedies offer safe, accessible ways to be proactive about your own health. You can use them for self-care when you get a cold, during bouts of insomnia, or to ease your digestion without worrying about serious side effects, overdose, or dependence. As long as you heed your doctor's advice about how to avoid unwanted interactions between natural remedies and any medications you're taking, an integrative approach to medicine that includes both paradigms is ideal.

Natural Remedies Increase Your Vitality

Conventional medicine defines health as an absence of disease. It has little to offer people who aren't suffering from an illness if they want to feel stronger, more energetic, or less susceptible to stress. This is where natural remedies shine! Certain preparations made from whole plants are known as tonics because they can increase vitality and enhance mental and physical performance. Traditional Chinese Medicine and Ayurveda have employed tonics to support longevity, fertility, immunity, and well-being for thousands of years, and scientific research proves that many of these traditional uses are valid. Beginning in the late 1940s with the work of Nikolai Lazarev, modern science dubbed many tonic herbs "adaptogens" for their ability to increase the body's resilience to all forms of stress. You'll find many recipes for tonics containing adaptogenic herbs (including ashwagandha, astragalus, eleuthero, and schisandra) in Chapters 7 and 8. Conventional medicine has nothing to offer with similar benefits.

Natural Remedies Are Cost-Effective

The benefits of using natural remedies would be enticing even if they came with a hefty price tag, but you don't need to spend a lot of money to experience the connection, creativity, and self-efficacy that comes from practicing natural self-care. Just like home cooking, home remedies are tastier and more cost-effective than their store-bought counterparts. Don't be seduced by the marketing in the supplement aisle. With very few exceptions (taking specific vitamins and minerals when you have a diagnosed deficiency, for example) the inexpensive remedies you can make at home will be better—and safer—than even the priciest mass-produced products you'll find at a health food store.

Natural Remedies Connect You to What Matters

The most important benefit of a natural, homemade approach to self-care is also the least obvious: it's a way to reconnect with the simple things that make life feel meaningful. Modern life is full of obstacles to nurturing authentic connections with each other, the land, and our own hearts. As a result, many people experience painful feelings of disconnection, isolation, and meaninglessness that have been proven to increase the risk of physical and mental illness. The act of making remedies and cooking healing foods is a powerful antidote for this distress. Every time you make one of the recipes in this book, you'll deepen your connections with Nature, the people you love, and your own creative spirit.

Simple Remedies Are Best

There's a lot of power in the little word *simple*. In Western folk herbalism "a simple" is a remedy made from a single plant chosen to match the specific needs of the person seeking relief. While not all of the remedies in this book are simples, the formulas throughout the book are as straightforward—and as simple!—as possible, using a minimal number of versatile ingredients. Once you've stocked your cabinets with herbs, essential oils, and natural ingredients, you'll be able to recombine them in nearly endless ways to create elegant solutions for a wide range of health needs.

An elegant solution achieves maximum effect with minimum effort. It's simple without cutting corners or dumbing things down. Scientists and mathematicians puzzle over a problem for years in order to find the simplest, most elegant solution. They follow a famous guideline called "Occam's razor." It goes something like this:

"All other things being equal, the simplest solution is best."

This guideline is similar to the way that modern medical science seeks the minimum effective dose for a course of treatment. Far from being lazy, the minimum effective dose is safest—and simplest. As different as the remedies in this book might be from scientific medicine, they share a commitment to the principles of simplicity and seeking the minimum effective dose. As you experiment with natural remedies and make decisions about how to take care of yourself, remember: the simplest solution is probably best.

Do Natural Remedies Work?

Plants are genius chemists. They rely on their ability to manufacture chemical compounds for every single aspect of their survival. A plant with juicy leaves can't run away to avoid being eaten. It relies on its own chemical defenses to kill microbes, deter pests, or poison would-be predators. Plants also need to reproduce. They can't impress a potential mate with a fancy dance, a victory in horn-to-horn combat, or a well-constructed nest like animals do. Since plants need to attract pollinators to accomplish sexual reproduction, they've evolved intoxicating scents, sweet nectar, and pheromones that send signals that bees and butterflies can't resist. When you consider that plants solve almost all of their problems by making chemicals, and that there are nearly 400,000 species of plants on Earth, it's no wonder that the plant kingdom is a source for a dazzling array of useful substances.

It's more than a sentimental notion to think of plants as our brothers and sisters. We grew up together over the millennia. At the same time that plants were evolving an amazing array of compounds and survival strategies, our animal ancestors were coevolving right alongside the plants. As plants developed their arsenal of phytochemicals (phyto = plant) to protect themselves from pests and predators, mammals developed the ability to use those same phytochemicals to their advantage. That's why so many of the chemicals that plants make for their own purposes have such beneficial effects on human health. For example, plants make chemicals that can:

- Relieve anxiety and depression
- Kill bacteria and fungi
- Combat viruses
- Stimulate the immune system
- Heal wounds
- Stop bleeding
- Restore normal heart rhythm
- Relieve pain
- Stimulate or sedate the central nervous system
- Affect hormone levels
- Relax muscle spasms
- Prevent cancer

If you drink tea or coffee to perk up, crave chocolate when you're sad or cranky, or eat fruits and veggies to stay healthy, you're already relying on the efficacy of plant compounds in your everyday life. The remedies in this book will teach you simple ways to extract beneficial compounds from a variety of helpful plants so you can harness their power. Our human ancestors were doing something similar before the start of recorded history. It worked for them, and it will work for you too.

Are Natural Remedies Safe?

You're on the right track if you're wondering about whether or not natural remedies carry risks of side effects, overdose, and dependence like pharmaceuticals. Your instinct might be telling you that anything that's powerful enough to heal is powerful enough to have the potential for harm. It's true. Natural remedies are no exception to this rule. The good news is that the risks of using natural remedies are low and easy to minimize if you apply common sense.

The most famous part of the Hippocratic Oath is also my rallying cry to anyone embarking on a self-care journey: first, do no harm. Whenever you reach for a remedy for yourself or someone you love, you're acting from one of the most beautiful aspects of human nature: compassion. It's a vital ingredient that supports healing, but it's not enough to ensure safety. Supplement your compassion with a protective dose of critical thinking by following the simple guidelines in the next section before you decide to use natural remedies. They'll help you differentiate when it's safe to take care of yourself at home and when you need to seek professional care.

Know When It's Safe to DIY

It's generally okay to use a home remedy when:

- Symptoms are mild.
- You are *not* running a high fever, having severe pain, having trouble breathing, or losing control of basic bodily functions.
- The situation is something that you could address with a trip to the drugstore for an over-the-counter remedy. Herbal remedies make great substitutes for many over-the-counter medications.
- Symptoms haven't been present for very long. This varies by condition, but generally if symptoms persist for two weeks, or worsen despite your self-care efforts, it's time to see a professional.

Always seek medical care in any of the following situations:

- Symptoms come on very quickly and/or are severe.
- You're experiencing chest pain or difficulty breathing.
- You have unexplained bleeding or bruising (including black tarry stools, blood on the toilet paper, or *any* vaginal bleeding after menopause).
- You've experienced unintentional, unexplained weight loss or notice a hard lump anywhere in your body that wasn't there before.
- Flu-like symptoms begin after you've traveled to a new locale, had sexual contact with a new partner, or gotten a bug bite.
- You're concerned that you might harm yourself or someone else. These are serious mental health symptoms that you should never ignore in yourself or in someone you love. Call 911 if necessary.

- You have a complex health history, have a chronic illness, or are taking medications that require close monitoring.
- Your intuition tells you that something is wrong. Even if you've seen a doctor before, if your intuition is nagging at you, don't ignore it.

When in doubt, seek qualified medical care. In many cases, the greatest harm you can do to yourself or your family is to delay obtaining a diagnosis until it's too late. Don't take that risk.

Know Yourself

Self-care is not a one-size-fits-all practice. Learning about yourself and your needs will point you toward the remedies in this book that will work best for you. Information about any illnesses you have, including the triggers that exacerbate your symptoms and any interventions that bring relief, will help you figure out how to take the best possible care of yourself. Your doctor and patient advocacy organizations can guide you toward trustworthy sources of information.

Know Your Family History

Knowing your family history is important too. If you know you're at higher risk for a certain condition, you can both prioritize the preventive measures most relevant to you and watch for warning signs so you can get treatment as quickly as possible if a problem starts to develop. For example, if there's a strong history of type 2 diabetes in your family, use that knowledge to motivate yourself to be proactive with good nutrition, regular exercise, and remedies like the Simplest Apple Cider Vinegar Tonic (see Chapter 6) to support balanced blood sugar. You can't do every single beneficial self-care practice, but you can apply your self-knowledge to help you choose the ones that will have the greatest impact.

Understand Your Medications

If you take medications, understanding how they work may help you to avoid potential interactions and side effects. The best general advice for avoiding herb/drug interactions is: don't treat a symptom with a home remedy and a pharmaceutical drug at the same time. (For example, don't use St. John's Wort along with prescribed antidepressants.) This book mentions some of the most common potential interactions for each remedy, but those lists are not exhaustive. Check with your doctor or pharmacist for personalized advice about which remedies are safe for you and which you should avoid.

If You're Pregnant and/or Nursing

Since there are strict ethical limits to conducting experimental research on pregnant women, patients and providers have to rely on less conclusive information about historical use, case studies, and in vitro research to make tentative determinations about the safety of herbs during pregnancy. Your choice to use any given remedy during pregnancy is a personal decision based on how you and your healthcare team evaluate the risks and benefits. While there are plenty of gray areas, a vast majority of herbalists and physicians agree that you should avoid the following during pregnancy:

- Remedies that cause strong intestinal or uterine contractions
- Remedies that affect hormone levels
- Remedies capable of bringing on a menstrual period
- Using any remedies during the first trimester unless advised to do so by a healthcare provider

The herbs mentioned in this book that are never safe during pregnancy are yarrow, mugwort, poke root, and red clover. Most essential oils are safe to use if they're diluted (at half the strength used for adults who aren't pregnant) in a carrier oil and applied to the skin. Aloe vera is safe to apply to your skin but not safe for internal use during pregnancy.

Many compounds in natural remedies can pass through breastmilk from mother to baby, just as compounds from food and medications do. Sometimes this can pose a serious risk to a developing baby. Other times it's possible to treat an issue that the baby is having by having the mother drink the appropriate remedies so she can pass them on to the infant through her breastmilk. An herbalist or midwife who specializes in women's health can help you to do this safely. To be on the safe side, avoid herbal remedies while nursing unless you've cleared them with your midwife, pediatrician, or other qualified practitioner.

Safety Guidelines for Children under Twelve

Many, but not all, of the remedies in this book are safe for children, but it's best to check with your pediatrician to be certain about what's appropriate for your child. Avoid giving children any of the stronger sedative herbs (skullcap, passionflower), any herbs with potential for side effects (lobelia), and remedies containing cayenne pepper, unless your practitioner recommends it and advises you how to adjust the dose. The topical remedies in this book are safe for children over one year of age as long as you dilute remedies containing essential oils to 50 percent of the strength recommended for adults. Lastly, remember never to give a remedy that contains honey to an infant under one year of age to prevent the risk of a rare but serious bacterial infection that only affects infants.

Safe and Effective Dosage

Except for a few plants (none of which are included in this book!), it's much more difficult to take a toxic dose of a plant-based medicine than of a pharmaceutical drug. The fiber, water, nutrients, and other components of whole plants dilute the concentration of any compounds that could prove dangerous if taken in large amounts. Our long evolutionary history of eating plants and using them for medicine has given us some built-in safeguards too. Most highly toxic plants taste bad. If a plant tastes terrible, or if your stomach feels queasy after taking a small amount, you'll automatically stop drinking or eating it! When you're working with safe plants, like the ones used in these recipes, the risk that you'll "overdose" is about as high as the risk of overdosing on spinach or blueberries—as long as you're following the other safety guidelines outlined in this chapter and any cautions listed for each remedy, of course.

All of the variables involved make herbal dosage more of an art than a science. The dosage instructions accompanying remedies in this book are guidelines to help you get started, not hard-and-fast rules, so don't be afraid to work your way up to large doses. For acute conditions, like anxiety or a cough, start with the dose recommended in the recipe, wait to see how you respond, and feel free to increase the next dose if you don't notice much improvement. For chronic conditions, like fatigue or acne, wait at least a week to see if your body responds before increasing the dose. If your symptoms worsen or persist for more than two weeks, it's best to discontinue natural remedies and consult a professional.

Learn Through Experience

There aren't any experts who can give you the gift of self-care. That particular power rests only with you. All of the benefits mentioned in this chapter are yours for the taking as soon as you put this book into practice.

The path to becoming an adept self-care practitioner resembles the path to becoming a confident cook. Get your hands and your heart involved in making something that appeals to you. Give yourself permission to make mistakes, and remember that mistakes sometimes lead to breakthrough discoveries. Make a recipe once or twice as it's written, then give yourself permission to experiment. You'll learn best by putting this knowledge into practice little by little, rather than trying to implement too many changes all at once. Just work your way through this book a little at a time and soon you'll have familiar routines that support all aspects of your health. The knowledge of how to care for yourself and your family with natural remedies can become an effortless part of your life, a reliable source of comfort that you can offer to yourself and the people you love. If you look back a few generations, you'll see that this knowledge has been part of your lineage before. Reclaiming these simple practices is your birthright. This book is just here to jog your memory.

Chapter 2

STOCKING UP

The quality of your homemade remedies depends on the quality of your ingredients. Whenever you're making a remedy, you're doing chemistry. Even the simplest cup of tea is technically a water extraction of herbal compounds; it can only taste good and offer medicinal benefits if the herbs are potent. Proper harvesting, processing, and packaging procedures yield high quality ingredients that will be easy for you to spot when you apply the knowledge in this chapter. Once you know how to identify trustworthy suppliers and high-quality ingredients, you'll be well on your way to making safe and effective remedies.

You can find many natural ingredients at your regular grocery store, though others will require a trip to a natural food store or a shop specializing in medicinal herbs. Even if you can't find everything you need locally, online suppliers (see my favorites in the Suppliers List in the Conclusion) make it easy to shop for everything you need. If you've never purchased bulk herbs or natural ingredients before, this chapter is all you need to demystify the process.

This chapter includes everything you need to know to stock up on the ingredients you'll need to make the recipes in this book. You'll learn how to tell a good-quality ingredient from one that's old, denatured, rancid, or weak; how to store and organize your remedies to maximize shelf life; and how to get the most value for your dollar when shopping for natural ingredients. A great way to approach this chapter is to choose a handful of recipes (no more than ten) you'd like to try and use them to create a shopping list. If you apply the knowledge from this chapter as you shop for that first batch of ingredients, the information will be more likely to stick. Besides, the sooner you source some ingredients, the sooner you'll get to the fun part—making remedies!

What to Have On Hand

Before you can stock up on supplies, you need to know what to look for and where to find it. This section will teach you how to find the fresh and dried herbs, carrier oils, tinctures, and essential oils featured in this book, as well as how to ensure that you're getting the best quality and value.

Grocery Store Basics

Shopping for natural ingredients at the grocery store is just like food shopping. Read labels and inspect your produce before purchasing and you'll be in great shape. Here are some pointers for specific ingredients used frequently in this book that you're likely to find at the grocery store:

- Basics like white vinegar, Epsom salt, and baking soda don't vary widely in quality. This is a good place to choose store-brand items to save money. Discount grocers and wholesale clubs stock these ingredients at an even greater savings. (You might be able to find extra-virgin olive and coconut oils there too!)
- Know what to look for in the produce aisle. Fresh herbs should be perky, green, and fragrant. Choose garlic bulbs that are tightly closed with the scraggly tips of their roots still attached. Best-quality fresh ginger has smooth skin; wrinkly skin is a sign that the root is old and dried out. Citrus fruit is protected by a thick skin, so it's safe to use conventionally grown citrus if you're only using the juice or the interior flesh. If you're going to be using the peel or the zest, choose organic citrus to avoid adding a serving of pesticides to your homemade remedies.
- Best-quality apple cider vinegar contains live cultures, sometimes called "the mother" of the vinegar. Bragg is the most famous brand, but any raw vinegar with the mother will work just as well.
- Be choosy about honey. Cheap honey might not be honey at all, in which case it won't have any medicinal properties. We're

facing an ecological crisis; beekeepers who care for their hives personally are doing a great service to all of us, so support local beekeepers whenever possible. Local honey has some additional benefits for you too. If you eat local honey year-round, it can help to reduce allergy symptoms during the spring.

- Miso paste is a traditional Japanese food that contains live cultures and provides beneficial probiotics in addition to its savory, salty flavor. Some grocery stores carry it, but you might have to go to a natural food store or Asian market to find it in your hometown. Make sure any miso you purchase is refrigerated (not powdered or freeze-dried) and is free from MSG. Miso Master (https://great-eastern-sun.com) and South River Miso (www.southrivermiso.com) are two of my favorite brands.

- Flaxseed comes in two forms: whole and ground. Whole seeds are your best bet. They stay fresh much longer, and you'll need them to make some of the recipes throughout the book. It you want the nutritional benefits of flaxseed as part of your regular diet, or to use it as an egg replacer in recipes, you can grind the whole seeds yourself. Use a small "bullet-style" blender or a coffee grinder dedicated to herbs and spices and grind in small batches for optimal freshness.

- Soy milk, almond milk, coconut milk, and other plant-based milks are widely available in grocery stores. Choose the unsweetened version of the plant milk you like best. Soy milk is richest in protein, which makes it creamy and great for frothy lattes. Almond milk is mild and low in calories. Coconut milk comes in two forms: canned (used most often in cooking) and in paper milk cartons for use as a beverage. For the recipes in this book, you can use any of these milks interchangeably except canned coconut milk, which cannot be substituted without altering the recipe significantly.

Remember that your local grocer is in business to please you. If she doesn't currently stock an ingredient you're looking for, you can request that she consider it. You might be surprised by how much influence you have. As more and more people embrace healthy lifestyles, natural ingredients that used to be specialty items will become easier to find in regular grocery stores.

Buying Bulk Herbs

The bulk bins of natural markets can be a great place to shop for the dried herbs you'll use to make teas and other remedies. If you don't have a natural market with bulk herbs in your town, you can order from a trusted online retailer like Mountain Rose Herbs (www.mountainroseherbs.com) or Frontier Co-op (www .frontiercoop.com/bulk-products/herbs/). Five Flavors Herbs (www.fiveflavorsherbs.com) in Oakland, California, stocks a wide range of bulk herbs, tinctures, and quality herbal products and will ship anywhere in the United States. I recommend them highly and use their pharmacy services to fill all of the custom formula orders for my clients. If you have an herb shop or health food store with a bulk herb section and want to try your hand at shopping for bulk herbs in person, here's what to look for:

- The colors should be bright and vibrant. Look for many different shades of green, lavender flowers that are distinctly purple, and chamomile flowers that are yellow. If all of the herbs look brownish and dull green, they're probably old and have lost much of their potency.
- Aromatic herbs should have strong, distinct, unmistakable odors. The best test for this is to contrast the smell of peppermint and spearmint. The difference should knock your socks off! If they smell pretty similar to each other, they're either very old or adulterated. Don't buy *anything* from a shop that has similar-smelling spearmint and peppermint.
- The company you're buying from should have a clear policy about conservation and protecting our medicinal plants from overharvesting and habitat destruction. United Plant Savers is a nonprofit organization dedicated to protecting the native medicinal plants of the United States and Canada. Make sure that any herbs on the United Plant Savers at-risk list (www .unitedplantsavers.org/species-at-risk) are cultivated, not harvested from the wild. (Echinacea is the only at-risk herb that's used in this book.)
- Be sure that herbs are labeled with both their common names and full Latin binomials. For example: lemon balm (*Melissa officinalis*).

While it's possible to make wonderful remedies with fresh herbs, dried herbs are easier to find, store, and work with when you're first getting started. Most of the remedies in this book are designed to work best with dried herbs. When a fresh herb is called for, it will either be a culinary herb (like rosemary or ginger) that you can find at the grocery store or a common medicinal weed that you can harvest yourself.

Purchasing Tea Bags and Tea Supplies

Blending and brewing loose-leaf and herbal teas is simple and rewarding when you have the equipment you need. When you don't want to craft your own remedy, or when you need a quick treat, premade tea bags are a convenient solution. Here's what you'll need to get the very best brew every time:

- **Teapot with a removable strainer:** Look for a teapot with a large strainer basket so that there's plenty of room for the water to circulate around the herbs, and make sure you can remove the strainer basket when the tea is done steeping. If you don't have a teapot, use a French press or a combination of two quart-sized Mason jars (one to brew the tea and a second to strain the tea into when it's done) and a fine-mesh strainer to get the job done.
- **Paper tea filters:** These are perfect for brewing single servings of herbal tea from dried herbs. Look for single-use filters that are compostable and designed to stand up on their own in your cup after you've opened them and added your herbs. You can also use a tea ball or a strainer spoon to brew single servings.
- **Teas:** Black, green, and white teas all come from the same plant: *Camellia sinensis.* (In fact, the only beverages that technically qualify as "tea" are the ones made from this plant. Herbal "teas" are properly called "tisanes.") The differences in flavor, antioxidant power, caffeine content, and price are all due to variations in how the leaves are harvested and processed. For the purposes of the recipes in this book, any black or green tea bags (including decaf) are sufficient as long as they don't contain any added flavors.

- **Check the label:** Are there any natural or artificial flavors listed in the ingredients? If so, avoid buying this product. Natural and artificial flavors interfere with your experience of the herbs in their natural state and aren't ideal for teas that you're using medicinally. If you're comfortable with natural and artificial flavors in your diet, it's okay to drink these teas just for enjoyment, but avoid using them for medicine.
- **For medicinal effect:** If you desire a medicinal effect from herbal tea bags, be sure to brew at double strength. (Laxative teas containing senna, rhubarb, or cascara sagrada are the exceptions to this rule!) Traditional Medicinals (www.traditionalmedicinals.com) is my favorite supplier of good-quality herbal tea bags.
- **Be wary:** Be wary of teas produced in China. As China has rapidly industrialized, many of the wonderful teas and herbs the country produces have been found to be contaminated with high levels of lead and other toxins.

Now that you've read this section, you know all the basics required to start experiencing the innumerable pleasures and benefits of regular tea drinking for yourself.

Shopping for Tinctures

Tinctures are herbal extracts made with alcohol. This book will teach you to make a few of your own, but since the process takes a minimum of three weeks and isn't ideal for all herbs, it's helpful to know how to shop for ready-made tinctures. Tinctures are convenient to use and have a much longer shelf life (one to five years, on average) than dried herbs and tea blends. Widely available brands that I recommend include Herb Pharm (www.herb-pharm.com) and Gaia Herbs (www.gaiaherbs.com); look for them in the "health and wellness" aisle at your local natural food store. If you don't need the tincture right away, Five Flavors Herbs and Herbalist & Alchemist (www.herbalist-alchemist.com) are wonderful suppliers that ship nationwide. If you're interested in buying your tinctures from another manufacturer, run these quality-control tests to suss out how well they know their stuff.

- If you can, check out a sample of the company's St. John's Wort tincture. It should be a deep ruby color. If it's not, something isn't right. I wouldn't buy from a manufacturer that can't make a potent tincture of St. John's Wort.
- Check the label of a bottle of *Lobelia inflata* tincture. If there isn't any vinegar or acetic acid in the bottle, don't buy anything from this company. Lobelia's active ingredients extract best in vinegar. If the company doesn't know that, I wouldn't trust them to effectively process other herbs either.
- If you avoid alcohol, look for extracts made with glycerin ("glycerites") or vinegar that are labeled "alcohol-free." Check the dosing instructions on the label before use since these preparations require different dosages than tinctures made from the same plant.

Tinctures can be applied directly to the skin, but they're most often taken by mouth. When taking a tincture orally, it's best to dilute it in water rather than squirting it directly into your mouth to protect your mouth and gums from the harshness of the alcohol. The amount of water you use is up to you. A tablespoon or two is enough, but if you find that the taste is still too strong, you can always use a full glass of water to dilute it further.

Finding Quality Carrier Oils, Butters, and More

Carrier oils and butters are fats used in herbal preparations to deliver beneficial plant compounds to the skin. In this book, you'll learn to use them to make infused oils and salves from fresh and dried herbs, to dilute essential oils for safe application, and to create luxurious homemade skincare products. Each carrier oil offers a unique set of properties. Some (coconut, olive, and sesame oils) are widely available in grocery stores, while others (jojoba oil and cocoa butter) are easier to find online or in natural food stores. No matter where you source your carrier oils, these tips will lead you toward the best of the bunch.

- The best oils are cold pressed. Avoid refined oils whenever possible.

- Delicate nut and seed oils can become rancid if they sit on the shelf too long or are exposed to high temperatures. Jojoba, olive, and unrefined sesame oils should have a delicate, round scent. Extra-virgin coconut oil should smell like coconuts! If an oil smells sharp or off-putting, it's likely rancid. Throw it away or return it to the store.

There are many more wonderful carrier oils and butters than the few included in this book. Feel free to experiment with a wide variety of carrier oils by following the substitution guidelines in the Conclusion whenever you try a new oil or butter for the first time. Don't be afraid to use a less expensive oil, like olive or sesame oil, to substitute for jojoba oil in recipes designed to be used on your hair and body.

Stocking Up on Essential Oils

Essential oils aren't true oils; they're delicate compounds that evaporate readily into the air and give each plant species its characteristic fragrance. These are potent ingredients that carry significant risks when used improperly. Treat them with respect and you'll find that essential oils are a joy to use, are easy to store, and offer delightful ways to perfume your home, enhance your mood, and combat microbes.

You'll learn more about essential oils and how to use them in Chapter 3, but be sure to stick to the following guidelines as you shop to make sure you're getting high-quality oils without adulterants or unreasonably high markups. After you educate yourself about what various oils look and smell like when they're well made, you'll be able to tell the difference.

- Do some homework on the manufacturer before you buy. Has the company been reprimanded by the FDA? Do they advocate unsafe practices, such as taking essential oils by mouth? If so, you shouldn't trust that company as a source of safe, unadulterated products.
- When companies use a process called gas chromatography to test and validate the chemical makeup of their essential oils, it indicates a high level of quality control. Responsible manufacturers often make gas chromatography reports available free

of charge to any customer who requests them. Check a company's website to see if it mentions this process, or email their customer service department to find out if they use it.

- Avoid buying essential oils from companies that use terms like *therapeutic grade*. There is no regulatory standard or certification process for such terms. The words are meaningless and misleading. Evaluate the oils and the company on the basis of other factors in this list.
- Reputable suppliers almost always package essential oils in dark glass bottles to protect them from light. Snow Lotus (www.snowlotus.org) is one trustworthy company that is an exception to this rule.
- Make sure that the listing for each oil includes the plant's Latin name (for example, *Lavandula officinalis* and *Lavandula angustifolia* are two different species of lavender), the country where it was harvested, and how it was extracted.
- Avoid essential oils extracted with hexane or other solvents since this process can hamper the essential oil's medicinal properties. Worse, the bottle may contain traces of solvents that could pose a health risk. The exception to this rule is rose absolute, which is safe to use when it comes from a reputable company.

The twelve oils described as follows are the only essential oils you'll need for the recipes in this book. They cover a wide range of applications so you can get most of the benefits of essential oils without spending a small fortune. Look for undiluted oils whenever possible, but be aware that rose, neroli, and lemon balm (and sometimes German chamomile) are usually sold already diluted in a carrier oil. These preparations are often wonderful; just avoid adding them to a diffuser or a water-based recipe.

Clary Sage (*Salvia sclarea*)
Relaxing and uplifting at the same time, clary sage calms the central nervous system without causing drowsiness. It has antispasmodic properties that can help to relax muscle tension, and its very mild estrogenic effect makes it especially useful for premenstrual syndrome and menopausal complaints. Just to be safe, avoid using clary sage if you have a history of estrogen-dependent cancer (such as breast cancer or ovarian cancer).

Geranium (*Pelargonium odoratissimum*)

With a versatile character and a pleasing fragrance reminiscent of the much more expensive rose oils, geranium is a great addition to your collection. Some people perceive it as relaxing, others as mildly stimulating. It's a wonderful addition to massage oils and to the bath, makes a great choice for home fragrance, and also has antifungal properties.

German Chamomile (*Matricaria recutita*)

Its gorgeous deep azure color is one of the clues to German chamomile's strength as an anti-inflammatory oil that shines in skincare applications. Calming, soothing, and cooling, this oil is a must-have for anyone with sensitive or troubled skin. It's also effective as a first aid treatment for minor burns, cuts, and scrapes.

Grapefruit (*Citrus paradisi*)

Like the other citrus oils, grapefruit is uplifting and refreshing. It has mild antimicrobial properties, which makes it well suited for use in homemade cleaning products, and I prefer it to lemon because it's a little bit unexpected. If you like the scent of lemon or orange better, you can substitute either of those oils in any recipes that call for grapefruit essential oil. All of the citrus oils can cause skin sensitivity, so avoid using them in skincare products—even when diluted.

Lavender (*Lavandula officinalis* or *Lavandula angustifolia*)

If you can buy only one essential oil, lavender is probably the best one to choose. It's wonderfully soothing and relaxing for the mind and nervous system, and it is an effective first aid for cuts, bug bites, minor burns, and skin irritations. When blended with other essential oils lavender has a harmonizing effect that helps "smooth out the rough edges" so that the blend comes together seamlessly.

Nutmeg (*Myristica fragrans*)

The haunting scent of nutmeg is as wonderful for home fragrance and body oils as it is in holiday treats. Nutmeg essential oil has mild pain-relieving properties, but its effects on the nervous system and the imagination are the ones that make it special. Diffusing nutmeg essential oil (see Chapter 3) is one of my favorite remedies for insomnia, and it makes a wonderful addition to aphrodisiac massage oils. At high doses (do not try this at home!) nutmeg has a hypnotic and hallucinogenic effect, as well as some significant safety risks. Small doses awaken the senses, calm the mind, and smell absolutely divine.

Peppermint (*Mentha piperita*)

Stimulating and uplifting, peppermint is one of the best essential oils for when you're feeling stuck and stagnant. Its cooling effect can bring welcome relief to headache sufferers, and it's also a great first aid for mild nausea and motion sickness.

Roman Chamomile (*Anthemis nobilis*)

As similar as their names may be, Roman chamomile essential oil has different effects and applications than German chamomile. Roman chamomile is profoundly antispasmodic and is one of the best oils to include in massage blends. It's also wonderfully soothing to the central nervous system and a great go-to oil for stress relief.

Rosemary (*Rosmarinus officinalis*)

Shakespeare's Ophelia made rosemary famous "for remembrance," and while it's useful as an aid for study and focus, its powers go much farther. When diffused or used in steam inhalation, rosemary can help relieve a bronchial infection by thinning the mucus and making it much easier for the body to expectorate. In skincare it's favored for its regenerating properties that help skin to heal and renew itself. Rosemary should not be used during pregnancy or by children under ten years of age.

Neroli (*Citrus aurantium*)

The tiny white flowers of the bitter orange tree produce this exquisite essential oil. It takes more than one hundred pounds of flowers to produce just one pound of essential oil, which is why neroli is one of the more expensive essential oils on the market and is often sold diluted in a carrier oil to make it more affordable. With its alluring fragrance that calms the mind and soothes emotional upset, in addition to benefits for rejuvenating the skin, I think a bottle of good neroli oil is worth every penny.

Lemon Balm (*Melissa officinalis*)

One of my favorite things to do is to watch a room of people inhale the fragrance of lemon balm for the first time. Within seconds, a sweet smile spreads across each person's face! There's no better essential oil to banish stress and lift your mood. Its sunny character makes lemon balm an ideal oil for people who experience a worsening of anxiety and depression symptoms during the winter. Lemon balm has antiviral properties and can help combat the herpes virus.

Rose (*Rosa damascena*) as Rose Absolute or Rose Otto

Rose is the queen of the flowers, not only because of her sumptuous appearance but also due to her fragrance and healing properties. Long associated with the heart, rose has antidepressant and antianxiety properties that are powerful enough to support people recovering from grief, trauma, or chronic illness. Since it takes a large volume of rose petals to produce a small amount of rose oil, you'll notice that the prices of rose oils are often much higher than those of other essential oils—even when diluted. Rose otto is produced by steam distillation and is the better choice for advanced skincare applications, but rose absolute is more affordable and is an appropriate choice for the recipes in this book.

Eat the Weeds

Here's a shocking fact: many of the most stubborn weeds that you battle in your yard and garden are actually medicinal plants! You can harvest them and use them as a source of fresh, local-as-it-gets wild food and medicine. So before you dig them up and throw them away or banish them with herbicides, check out some of the remedies that you can make with common weeds. Here are some pointers to remember when harvesting weeds:

- Avoid plants that have been sprayed with herbicides or pesticides.
- Avoid harvesting weeds that are growing within 1 foot of the curb on a residential or side street, or within 5 feet of a highway. If you avoid gathering weeds near sidewalks, the chances that a dog peed on your harvest are pretty slim. And if you stay away from the highway, you'll avoid pollution from runoff and the risk of an accident.

- Wash your harvest the same way you'd wash produce from the grocery store. Allow the plants to dry *completely* before using them in recipes for salves or infused oils since even a little bit of water on the leaves could cause your finished product to spoil rapidly.

With a little practice, you'll start spotting these medicinal weeds everywhere—even when you're not looking! Here are some pointers to help you find your first few harvests:

- Dandelion (*Taraxacum officinale*): Look in lawns, fields, gardens, and even cracks in the sidewalk. Toothed leaves, yellow flowers, and a long taproot are key identifying characteristics for dandelion. It's easy to harvest leaves and flowers by hand, but you'll need a straight trowel or root-digging tool to harvest the taproots.
- Plantain (*Plantago* spp.): This isn't the starchy fruit that looks like a banana! It's a medicinal weed that's a powerhouse for healing skin and other epithelial tissue. Look for this plant on playgrounds, paths, and other places where the soil has been packed down by heavy foot traffic. *Plantago lanceolata* has skinny leaves, while *Plantago major* has thick leaves that taper at the ends. Both species are medicinal and have leaves with parallel veins organized in a basal rosette. Harvest by hand and use it either fresh or dried in many recipes in this book, including Luxurious Toner for All Skin Types (see Chapter 4); First Aid Salve with Yarrow, Calendula, and Plantain (see Chapter 4); and Herbal Mouthwash (see Chapter 6).
- Poke root (*Phytolacca americana*): This impressive weed grows throughout the United States and is most prevalent in the South. It grows best in disturbed ground, often at the borders between wild spaces and mowed lawns or near run-off streams. Look for a tall plant with broad leaves and blackish purple berries that stain bright pink. Harvest the roots in the fall after the first frost. You'll need a serious shovel!

Once you start building your collection of herbs and natural ingredients, you're going to need a system to keep them fresh and organized.

How to Store and Organize Your Remedies and Ingredients

Unpacking a big box full of bulk herbs, butters, and natural ingredients is lots of fun, but figuring out how to fit a bunch of irregularly shaped bags, bottles, and tubs into your cupboards without displacing your dishes or pantry supplies may take a little bit of trial and error. It's worth investing some time to come up with a storage system that covers the remedy-making process from start to finish. No matter how you design your system, you'll want to ensure that the equipment and ingredients you need for remedy making are accessible, that there's a place to store supplies for bottling and labeling your creations, and that your finished remedies are stored to maximize shelf life in a place where you'll remember to use them.

Here are some tips to make storage and organization easier:

- Clear a dedicated space to prevent clutter. Choose a spot that's protected from sunlight and extreme temperatures.
- If you don't have room to clear a shelf or cupboard, use stackable clear plastic bins instead. (I use "shoe storage" bins from The Container Store.) They'll protect your ingredients, and the clear plastic makes it easy to find the right bin when you need it.
- Avoid storing ingredients in the bathroom. Temperature and humidity fluctuations in the bathroom can cause spoilage. Keeping finished remedies that you use daily (skincare, witch hazel pads, etc.) in the bathroom is okay. Just don't use it as a spot for long-term storage.
- Consider repurposing a small train case, makeup carrier, or other portable container to store your essential oils. Bottles of essential oils are small and portable, which also makes them easy to lose track of. If you keep all of your oils together in a portable kit, you'll always know where to find them and you'll be able to bring them with you to any room of the house where you'd like to use them.

Last, but certainly not least, label everything! There is no possible way for me to overemphasize this! You might like to store finished remedies in the same place as your ingredients, or they might feel like a more natural fit in the cabinet with vitamins, over-the-counter medicines, and supplements. Whether you're storing leftover tea in the fridge for a day, stocking the freezer with herb-infused broth, or putting a finished tincture in a cupboard, the label you put on the container is the most important part of your storage system.

If you're like most people I know, the day will come when you've whipped up a fresh batch of Chocolate Spice Bitters or Sensual Ginger and Coconut Massage Oil and you'll think, *I don't need to label this.* Maybe you're out of labels, maybe you don't have any other bottles that look similar, or maybe you think you'll be able to easily identify the contents by scent alone. If you give in to this temptation, know that the time will come when you won't remember what's in that bottle and, when that happens, you'll have no choice but to toss a perfectly good remedy. Labels don't have to be fancy to be effective; even a strip of masking tape will do as long as it includes the right information.

Labels should always include:

- The name of the finished remedy
- The date you bottled it
- A list of ingredients used, ideally in descending order by volume
- Important safety information ("for external use only," for example), if applicable

Keep a sheet of labels, a permanent marker, and/or some pretty tape (I use Japanese washi tape) in the same place where you keep your ingredients so labeling is a breeze.

Now that you've learned a little bit about how natural remedies work and know what to look for when gathering ingredients and supplies, there's only one thing left to do: try some recipes! Remember: your own experience will be your best teacher.

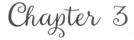

Chapter 3

THE
HEALTHY
HOME

It's easier to eat well when your fridge is stocked with fresh fruits and veggies, and it's easier to exercise if you set out your workout clothes before you go to bed so they're waiting for you in the morning. Creating a supportive environment is one of the smartest steps you can take toward achieving your goals. The same principle applies to practicing a wellness-centered lifestyle. If you want to feel healthier, happier, and more relaxed, start with your home. Your living space has a tremendous impact on your well-being.

In this chapter you'll learn how plants, essential oils, and natural ingredients can help you to turn your home into a supportive sanctuary. You'll also find plenty of ideas to bring beauty and coziness to your space so you can relax and feel nurtured. Before you know it, you'll be reaping the benefits of air-purifying houseplants, sweet-smelling potpourri, and essential oil blends to suit any mood. An array of homemade cleaning products will help you save money and avoid buying toxic chemicals too. Once you see how effective, affordable, and luxurious it is to use herbs and natural ingredients around the house, I hope you'll be emboldened to venture deeper into this book.

Health-Promoting Houseplants

Have you ever noticed that when you take a walk through the woods or a garden, the simple presence of trees, fresh air, and flowers calms you down? Modern life requires most of us to spend our time indoors, but houseplants make it possible to bring some of the benefits of living plants into your home and office. The plants in this section are easy to care for, improve indoor air quality, and make any space feel a little more tranquil.

⊷ Aloe Vera ⊶

BENEFITS AND USES: *provides instant first aid for minor cuts, scrapes, and burns; beautifies your home; and purifies the air*

AVOID: *ingesting; leaving within reach of dogs and cats (aloe is toxic for them)*

YIELDS: ½–5 tablespoons depending on leaf size

➤ **1 fresh aloe vera leaf**

1 *To harvest aloe vera gel:* Using a sharp knife, cut the leaf you want to harvest from the stalk of the plant, making your cut as close to the stalk as you can. Rinse the leaf and pat dry.

2 Look for the yellow sap at the cut edge of the aloe vera leaf. Cut off the part of the leaf with the highest concentration of this yellow sap—usually about ½"–1" from the base. This sap contains an irritant (aloin) that the plant uses to protect itself. Your finished product will be best if it has as little aloin in it as possible.

3 Cut the spines off of the leaf so that you won't cut yourself while working. Then cut the leaf into 2"–3" sections.

4 Trim away the rind from the sticky, solid gel at the center of the leaf with a knife. Apply to affected areas for first aid or use in skincare recipes. Store leftover gel in the refrigerator inside a nonreactive container (glass and heavy plastic are fine; avoid metal containers) covered with a lid up to 3 days. If you want to store the gel longer than 3 days, freeze it using the following directions.

5 *To freeze fresh aloe vera gel:* After removing the gel from the leaves, place it in a blender and process on high until liquefied, about 1 minute in a high-speed blender or up to 3 minutes in a standard blender.

6 Pour blended aloe vera gel into an ice cube tray and freeze until solid.

7 Pop cubes of gel out of the tray and store in a freezer bag to preserve their freshness. Use within 6 months.

Peace Lily

BENEFITS AND USES: *helps with air purification*

AVOID: *if you have dogs or cats who are likely to eat your houseplants (peace lilies are toxic for them)*

YIELDS: 1 room of cleaner air

➤ **1 peace lily plant**

1 Pot a new peace lily in potting soil designed for houseplants, making sure to add 1"–2" of rocks at the bottom of the pot before adding your soil to ensure good drainage. Most peace lilies will be potted appropriately when you buy them, but follow these instructions if you need to repot after a few years of growth.

2 Give your peace lily access to plenty of natural light during the spring and summer months, and provide access to low light during fall and winter. Changing the light with the seasons will help your plant to bloom and grow, but your plant can live in low light year-round if necessary.

3 Water regularly enough to prevent the plant from wilting. In a hot, dry climate this could be as often as daily, while in a humid, temperate climate you might need to water only once per week. You can avoid overwatering by making sure that the top inch or two of soil has time to dry out between waterings. Once the soil is dry, it's safe to water again.

4 If your home is very dry during the winter months, your peace lily can suffer wilting and stunted growth. To avoid this, mist the leaves with a spray bottle filled with water or, once a week, put your plant into your bathtub and let the shower spray cool or room temperature (not hot!) water on the whole plant and its container for a minute or two. Then leave the plant in the shower (with the water turned off) for the next eight to twelve hours so that it can bask in the leftover humidity.

✴ Spider Plant ✴

BENEFITS AND USES: *helps with air purification*

AVOID: *N/A*

YIELDS: 1 room of cleaner air

➤ **1 spider plant "baby"**

1   The best way to obtain a spider plant is to ask for one or two "spider-ettes" or "babies" from a friend with a mature plant. Mature plants send out shoots with tiny "baby" plants attached. These mini-plants will grow into full sized spider plants and go on to produce "babies" of their own.

2   To pot a baby spider plant, cut the baby from the mature plant. Look at the underside of the baby plant for a root bundle. Plant root-side down in a pot with potting soil designed for houseplants.

3   Keep your spider plants out of direct sunlight. They'll be happiest in moderate light.

4   Allow any "babies" to grow to about 2" in size before repotting them.

5   Water spider plants regularly. You'll need to water more often in a hot, dry climate or if you use very small pots that dry out quickly. The best way to know how often to water is to watch the soil. If you allow the soil to dry out completely between waterings, you'll never overwater.

 remedy notes

An air-purifying wunderkind, spider plants remove the toxic compounds xylene and toluene from the air. They also produce lots of "babies" so you can spread the air-purifying love to multiple rooms of the house and to friends and family members. Spider plants are nontoxic to cats and dogs, too, so this plant is a great choice if you don't trust your animals not to chew on a houseplant from time to time.

Herbal Potpourris

It might seem antiquated to blend your own potpourri, but if you try it once, the pleasures of the process will convince you that it's worth your time. Using potpourri is the best way to impart a fragrance to your whole house (use the stovetop method described in the recipes for this effect), and the blends you create can also work beautifully in sachets or set out in pretty dishes. However you choose to enjoy your finished blends, you'll be using the power of fragrance to speak directly to the emotional center of the brain. With these simple recipes, you can enhance mood, create a sense of safety, and help support better sleep—all without any risks of herb/drug interactions, unpleasant taste, or side effects.

Lavender Rose Potpourri

BENEFITS AND USES: *creates a calming, grounding atmosphere in your home*

AVOID: *N/A*

YIELDS: about 3½ cups

- 1 cup dried lavender flowers
- 1 cup dried rose petals
- 1 cup dried red clover
- ½ cup powdered orris root
- ¼ cup whole cloves
- 5 drops nutmeg essential oil
- 5 drops geranium essential oil
- 4 cups water

1 Stir together all ingredients except water in a large bowl. Store in a covered jar up to 3 months until ready to use.

2 To use, simmer water and 1 cup of the finished mixture on the stove to give a beautiful fragrance to the whole house. Or, for a gentler experience, set out the potpourri in small dishes to impart subtle fragrance to any room. You could also enclose it in sachets to add fragrance to drawers where you store your clothing.

remedy notes

The orris root used in this recipe comes from two species of iris and is available in many craft stores and through the same bulk herb suppliers mentioned in Chapter 2. It contributes a deep base note to the fragrance, and also serves as a fixative to help the potpourri keep its fragrance longer. Cinnamon sticks can serve as fixatives, too, and are the best substitute if you don't have any orris root on hand.

Sleepytime Potpourri

BENEFITS AND USES: *helps with deep relaxation and better sleep*

AVOID: *using near cats*

YIELDS: 3¼ cups

> 1 cup dried chamomile flowers

> 1 cup dried lavender flowers

> ½ cup dried red clover

> ½ cup dried mugwort

> ¼ cup powdered orris root

> 5 drops lavender essential oil

> 5 drops Roman chamomile essential oil

> 4 cups water

---

1 Stir together all ingredients in a large bowl. Store in a covered jar up to 3 months until ready to use.

2 To use, place potpourri in small dishes in the bedroom, tuck it into small sachets that will fit inside your pillows, or use it to fill an herbal dream pillow (a small pillow stuffed with potpourri that you keep nearby when sleeping). You can also simmer water and 1 cup of the blend in an uncovered pot, but make sure that you don't fall asleep with the burner on!

 remedy notes

Chamomile and lavender create a synergistic blend; their combined relaxation-inducing power is stronger than when either herb is used on its own. Mugwort has many medicinal uses, but this blend draws upon its folk reputation for bringing sweet dreams and protecting your spirit so you can let go and sleep deeply.

Apple Cinnamon Potpourri

BENEFITS AND USES: *induces feelings of warmth, safety, and comfort*

AVOID: *N/A*

YIELDS: about 2½ cups

- 1 cup dried apple slices, tightly packed
- ½ cup dried sage leaves
- ½ cup dried bay leaves
- ¼ cup whole cloves
- ⅛ cup fresh orange zest
- 6 cinnamon sticks
- 4 cups water

1 Add all ingredients except water to a large bowl and toss with your hands until combined. Store in a covered jar up to 1 month until ready to use.

2 To use, simmer water and 1 cup of the finished mixture on the stove to give a beautiful fragrance to the whole house.

remedy notes

Feeling safe is the first step toward healing, and this blend can help you feel grounded, centered, and supported. Whenever you feel safe and comfortable, your parasympathetic nervous system is better able to do its important work of "resting and digesting." Don't underestimate the healing power of the comforting, cozy feelings this blend evokes; they're a signal that you're maximizing your capacity for self-healing!

✦ Sweet Petal Lingerie Drawer Liners ✦

BENEFITS AND USES: *repels pests*

AVOID: *N/A*

YIELDS: 1 drawer liner

> **Cotton fabric (see step 1 for measurement instructions)**
> **1 heaping cup dried lavender flowers**
> **2 drops geranium essential oil**
> **Double-sided fabric tape**

1 Before starting this project, measure the length and width of the bottom of each drawer that you would like to line. Double the measurement to find the amount of fabric you'll need for each drawer. For example, if the bottom of your drawer measures 22" × 15", you'll need to buy 2 yards of fabric or find two pieces of scrap fabric that are at least 22" × 15".

2 Cut two identical pieces of fabric to fit just inside the measurements of your drawer. You want the fabric to be ever so slightly smaller (about ⅛" on each side) than the inside of the drawer to prevent the liner from bunching up.

3 Place dried lavender flowers into a clean mixing bowl. Add geranium essential oil and toss gently with your fingers to evenly distribute.

4 Lay your identical pieces of fabric on your work surface so that the wrong side of each piece of fabric is facing up. Apply double-sided fabric tape to three sides of one piece of fabric, leaving one short side without tape. Align the matching piece of fabric on top, wrong side down. Peel the paper off the double-sided tape and affix the second piece of fabric over the first to create a "pocket" that's closed on three sides and open on one short side.

Sweet Petal Lingerie Drawer Liners—continued

5 Add a single layer of geranium-scented lavender flowers to the inside of the fabric "pocket" you've created. When you're satisfied with the amount of flowers in the middle, close the open side of the liner by applying a final piece of double-sided fabric tape to the wrong side of the fabric and pressing the pieces together to affix.

6 Place the liner inside the drawer. Use your hands to smooth out any lumps, but don't worry about making it perfectly smooth. If desired, you can apply a small square of double-sided tape to each corner of the liner to help it stay in position.

7 When the fragrance fades, pull apart the double-sided tape on one side to open the liner. Then replace the spent flowers with a fresh batch and reseal with a new piece of tape.

These liners are wonderful for sweater drawers and off-season clothing storage! For a more elegant construction, sew the liners on three sides and close the final side of the pocket with Velcro or a hook-and-loop-style product. You can experiment with other dried flowers (rose petals or jasmine flowers would both be lovely) and essential oils too.

✦ Orange Clove Pomanders ✦

BENEFITS AND USES: *deters pests and helps decorate your home*

AVOID: *placing within reach of pets and toddlers*

YIELDS: 1 pomander

> 1 medium orange (approximately 5" in diameter)

> ⅛ cup whole cloves

1 Press as many whole cloves into the skin of the orange as possible, making sure that no more than ¼" of bare orange skin remains between each clove. (If your thumb gets sore from pressing the cloves into the orange skin, use a thimble to protect it.)

2 Once you've covered the entire orange with cloves, place the pomander in your cupboard to keep ants and other pests away, in your closet to deter moths, or in a decorative bowl for room fragrance. You can also tie two ribbons around the orange to turn the pomander into a hanging ornament. First, lay down two decorative ribbons on your work surface in a cross pattern. Center the pomander over the place where the ribbons cross one another and tie each ribbon around the pomander so that it's held securely. Then tie the hanging ornament to a sturdy garland or banister you'd like to decorate.

remedy notes

Making pomanders has therapeutic benefits. Pomander making is a great stress-relieving activity during the holiday season for both kids and adults. Piercing the orange's skin with the cloves releases the essential oil into the air and its fragrance helps to calm the mind and body. Orange essential oil has been shown to reduce symptoms of post-traumatic stress disorder and relieve depression. When you're done, you'll have beautiful little creations that you can use for holiday decorations or as nontoxic pest deterrents anywhere in the house.

Essential Oils

Essential oils aren't really oils at all; they're aromatic compounds that evaporate quickly and give each plant species its characteristic fragrance. In this section you'll get to know the properties of each oil and practice combining oils into novel blends that will delight your senses. The best way to get started with essential oils is to use them in a diffuser designed to emit a fine mist of diluted essential oil (or blends) into the air. Perfuming your home with diffused essential oils has medicinal benefits that go beyond the pleasures of fragrance. Diffusing oils that lift the mood, reduce stress, and promote concentration is a great approach to supporting emotional and mental health at home. Oils with antimicrobial properties can relieve sinus issues and prevent airborne germs from spreading through your space. They're so powerful that just one or two drops, used properly, can make a big difference in your day.

Choose Your Oils

Think about what you want your oil to accomplish. Do you want it to uplift your spirits, help you calm down and get ready to fall asleep, or combat the germs of a sneezing family member? You don't have to memorize the functions of each essential oil if you keep this general principle in mind: the part of the plant the volatile oil comes from can help you predict its function. Essential oils that come from flowers (rose, geranium, neroli) are the plant's way of enticing pollinators to come closer. Their sweet fragrances are just as appealing to us as they are to bees, and they tend to have beneficial effects on our mental processes, hormones, and moods with comparatively little antimicrobial activity. Oils that come from leaves and bark, however, are more likely to be part of the plant's self-defense system. These oils may repel pesky insects, fight fungal infections, and have potent antibacterial and antiviral activity. Now that you have a general framework for understanding what essential oils can do for you, it's time to start experimenting!

Start with Simples

The easiest way to learn the benefits and properties of essential oils is through a combination of research and personal experience. At first you'll need to consult this book to figure out which oils are best for the uses you have in mind, but your personal experience with each oil will be the best teacher of all. The best way to develop a working knowledge of essential oils with minimal time and effort is to start by using your oils one at a time as *simples*. Any herbal preparation made from a single plant is called a simple.

Preparing a simple is, well…simple! After you decide what you want to accomplish with your oil, consult the descriptions in Chapter 2 to choose one that seems well suited to your goal, then diffuse it on its own using the instructions given later in this chapter. Notice how it affects you. Does it seem cooling (like peppermint) or warming (like rosemary)? Is it relaxing or energizing? You might even like to keep some notes about how each oil smells, how it makes you feel physically, and what effects it has on your mind and spirit. This will help you get to know each plant's personality and effects direct from the source. If you repeat this process with all of the essential oils mentioned in this book, you'll be well on your way to mastering the skills needed to create your own customized blends and formulas.

Pairings and Triads

Once you're familiar with the individual oils, try pairing two oils together. Like two close friends or a married couple, two herbs are often better than one. They can balance each other out and create something better than the sum of their parts. Triad formulas are a little more complex, but once you try your hand at the ones I've suggested in the following list, you'll be ready to experiment with your own novel combinations.

- **Lavender and Peppermint:** Lavender is relaxing and peppermint is stimulating, but both have a cooling "energy." The contrast of the calming and stimulating effects makes this blend excellent for stress relief during the daytime, and it's an especially powerful combination for headaches. *Formulation principle:* combining herbs with opposite effects (stimulation and relaxation) and similar energetics (cooling) can be a great way to untangle stress without becoming sleepy.
- **Peppermint and Tea Tree:** Peppermint's antimicrobial powers pale in comparison to tea tree's, but tea tree lacks the sweet

charm and uplifting scent that makes peppermint so pleasant. Combining the two makes for a much more enjoyable antimicrobial experience than tea tree can offer on its own. *Formulation principle:* when one herb doesn't smell or taste so great, add a pleasing one to make the experience more enjoyable without losing any therapeutic benefits.

- **Geranium and Nutmeg:** Both of these oils have haunting, enticing aromas. Geranium comes from the flowering parts of the plant, while nutmeg comes from the seed and has a much heavier quality. The lightness of the floral note (geranium) is balanced by the depth of the base note (nutmeg), and the combination is a wonderful aphrodisiac blend. Experiment with both an equal ratio and a 2:1 ratio of geranium to nutmeg and vice versa for a great lesson in balancing the "weight" of a fragrance. *Formulation principle:* balance lighter floral oils with heavier notes from seeds, barks, and roots.
- **Roman Chamomile, Rosemary, and Geranium:** This blend provides the depth and sweetness of two floral oils (Roman chamomile and geranium) that encourage muscle relaxation and hormonal balance with an uplifting kick from the rosemary. Notice the way that using two similar oils with one contrasting oil creates effects that are so different from using each oil on its own. *Formulation principle:* create a complex blend by combining two oils with similar properties with one contrasting oil.
- **Grapefruit, Clary Sage, and Rosemary:** All three of these oils have uplifting and antimicrobial properties, but the contrast between the citrus oil and the herbaceous oils makes the blend really sing. Try 5 drops of grapefruit with 2 drops each of clary sage and rosemary. *Formulation principle:* diversify a blend by choosing oils with similar properties that come from different parts of a plant or different kinds of plants.
- **Rosemary, Peppermint, and Tea Tree:** This is a powerhouse blend for the respiratory tract. Rosemary and tea tree boast serious antimicrobial power, while peppermint opens the sinuses so that the other two oils can have maximum impact. This is a perfect blend for summertime colds and sinus infections. *Formulation principle:* combine two oils with strong therapeutic effects with a small amount of a third oil (try a 4:1 ratio as follows: 2 drops each rosemary and tea tree with 1 drop peppermint) that "guides" the blend to the part of the body that needs support.

⊹⊱ Essential Oil Diffusers ⊰⊹

BENEFITS AND USES: *helps with home fragrance, stress relief, and respiratory health*

AVOID: *if you have cats, dogs, or birds in your house, unless the oil you're using is safe for your animal*

YIELDS: about 2–4 hours of treatment

- 1 diffuser designed for use with essential oils
- Water per manufacturer's instructions
- 5–15 drops of your chosen essential oils (Note: essential oils diluted in a carrier oil will *not* work in a diffuser.)

1 Fill the diffuser with the amount of water specified by the manufacturer's instructions.

2 Add 5–15 drops of essential oils. The proper dose depends on the size of the water reservoir in your diffuser and the intended purpose of the oils. Consult the manufacturer's instructions for the specific amount of essential oil that's ideal for your unit. Avoid using too much essential oil at one time to prevent irritation.

3 Secure the lid and turn on the diffuser. Allow it to run for the desired length of time.

4 Clean the diffuser after each use. Empty any remaining water from the reservoir, rinse with clean water, and wipe dry with a clean cloth. Allow the unit to dry thoroughly to prevent mold or mildew.

remedy notes

If you have pets, do not use essential oils in any indoor environment that your animal shares without consulting your veterinarian first. Even small amounts of exposure to the wrong oils can be fatal to cats, dogs, and birds.

All-Natural Cleaning Products

When your home smells fresh and the surfaces are sparkling clean, it's easier to relax and unwind. Being in a clean environment just feels better. Cleaning products can help make the job easier, but many of the cleansers you can buy at the store are full of strong chemicals that can irritate your skin and respiratory system, cause sensitivities, disrupt your hormones, promote the growth of antibiotic-resistant bacteria, and harm the environment. The good news is that you don't have to choose between a clean house and a natural lifestyle. The homemade cleansers in this section will give you the sparkling clean surfaces and fresh scents that make your space look and feel great—without any harsh chemicals. The ingredients are safe and inexpensive, and the recipes couldn't be easier. In fact, they almost make cleaning *fun*!

Clary Sage and Tea Tree Shower Spray

BENEFITS AND USES: *prevents mold and mildew in the bathroom*

AVOID: *if you're sensitive to any of the ingredients—especially the scent of vinegar*

YIELDS: 1½ cups

- 1 cup water
- ½ cup white vinegar
- 4 drops tea tree essential oil
- 4 drops clary sage essential oil

1 Combine all ingredients in a plastic spray bottle that can hold at least 12 ounces of fluid.

2 Shake well for 15 seconds before each use.

3 Spray liberally on areas that are prone to mildew. Let sit 3–5 minutes and wipe dry.

remedy notes

Vinegar is a gentle cleansing agent that's safe to use on tile, glass, and grout. Tea tree essential oil is a powerful antifungal ingredient that's effective against mold and mildew. If your shower has a mold or mildew problem, try applying tea tree essential oil directly to the affected areas before scrubbing or scouring. Repeat a few times per week until the mildew is gone. Be careful not to get undiluted essential oil on your hands.

Coconut Oil Wood Polish

BENEFITS AND USES: *rehabs dried-out wood furniture or helps polish solid wood pieces that haven't been sealed or varnished*

AVOID: *using on pressed wood. Always test a small amount in an inconspicuous place on the piece of furniture you're going to be working on before applying a large amount.*

YIELDS: ⅛ cup

> ⅛ **cup coconut oil**
> **1 microfiber cloth**

1 Scoop coconut oil into a microwave-safe bowl. Warm oil by microwaving it 15 seconds at a time and stirring after each 15-second interval until it liquefies.

2 Dab a microfiber cloth into liquefied oil.

3 Rub oil into furniture, using a very small amount for each piece.

remedy notes

If you're working with wood that's old, distressed, or in need of TLC, you can add more oil and rub it into the wood until it's absorbed. If the piece is very large, very old, or in rough shape, it might absorb much more than ⅛ cup of oil, so you may need to make a second batch. Store any leftovers in a covered, labeled container at room temperature. Keep the container out of your pets' reach and separate from coconut oil that you use for cooking and/or skincare.

Flowers and Spice Floor Wipes

BENEFITS AND USES: *cleans tile and linoleum flooring; can also be used occasionally on sealed hardwood floors*

AVOID: *using on unsealed hardwood flooring*

YIELDS: 2 cups (enough for about 5 cloths)

- 1 cup water
- 1 cup white vinegar
- 5 drops nutmeg essential oil
- 5 drops geranium essential oil
- 5 drops lavender essential oil
- 5 cellulose cloths, size 7" × 7" or 7.5" × 10"
- Electrostatic mop

1. Combine water, white vinegar, and essential oils in a small mixing bowl. Stir to combine.

2. Soak cellulose cloths in vinegar mixture 2–3 minutes, until much of the liquid is absorbed. After the initial soak, you can use the wipes right away or store them in a plastic tub or zip-top bag up to 6 months. If storing, make sure to include any leftover fluid in the container to keep the wipes moist.

3. To use the wipes, remove a single wipe from the tub or zip-top bag. Lightly wring out excess liquid. Attach wipe to any electrostatic mop and run over floors. After one side becomes soiled, turn over the wipe, reattach it to the mop, and use the other side.

4. After use, the cloths can be cleaned, stored, and reused. Most cellulose cloths can be run through the dishwasher or washing machine. Check the packaging for instructions on cleaning and reuse.

 remedy notes

The vinegar is the most important cleansing agent in this recipe. Since the essential oils are primarily for fragrance, feel free to experiment with any combination of oils that you enjoy. Keep in mind that vinegar can dull hardwood over time, so use this mixture no more than once or twice per month on hardwood floors. Use as often as desired on linoleum or tile.

✦ Grapefruit Rosemary ✦
Sink and Tub Scrub

BENEFITS AND USES: *helps with weekly or biweekly cleaning*

AVOID: *using on aluminum*

YIELDS: 1 cup

- **1 cup baking soda**
- **3 drops rosemary essential oil**
- **3 drops grapefruit essential oil**

---

1 Combine all ingredients in a small plastic tub. (You can use a Tupperware container for this or recycle a plastic container. At my house, I use empty miso paste containers—they're the perfect size!)

2 Stir with a fork to distribute essential oils throughout baking soda. If you're not using the cleanser right away, close the container with the lid and store out of the reach of pets and small children. The cleanser won't go bad, but the fragrance will dissipate after 3 months.

3 To use, sprinkle 1–2 tablespoons cleanser into the sink or ½ cup into the tub. Scrub thoroughly with a wet sponge, adding more cleanser as needed.

4 Rinse thoroughly with water to reveal sparkling clean surfaces.

remedy notes

This is a great way to de-grunge a sink! While it boasts antimicrobial properties and smells fantastic, this cleanser is not a full-spectrum disinfectant. If you need to disinfect a sink that has come into contact with raw meat, bodily fluids, or germs from someone with a contagious disease, a formula containing bleach is your safest bet. Baking soda is mildly abrasive, so test a small area first if you're unsure about using this recipe on any particular piece.

✈ Tea Tree Toilet Bowl Cleanser ✈

BENEFITS AND USES: *helps with weekly or biweekly cleaning to lightly disinfect and scrub the toilet bowl*

AVOID: *using on a toilet that's been used by someone with a contagious disease; use bleach instead*

YIELDS: enough to clean one toilet bowl

> **5 drops tea tree essential oil**
> **¼ cup baking soda**
> **⅛ cup white vinegar**

1 Drop 5 drops tea tree essential oil into the toilet bowl.

2 Sprinkle baking soda evenly over the inside of the toilet bowl, avoiding the water as much as possible.

3 Scrub with toilet brush to remove any visible marks, stains, or mildew.

4 Pour vinegar over the inside of the toilet bowl and watch it fizz.

5 Scrub once more with the toilet brush until the toilet bowl is sparkling clean. Flush.

remedy notes

For increased antimicrobial effects between cleanings, add 1–2 drops of tea tree oil to the toilet bowl and let stand until the next time the toilet is flushed after use.

Naturally Fragrant DIY Dryer Sheets

BENEFITS AND USES: *gives your clothes the clean, fresh scent of your choice without any synthetic chemicals*

AVOID: *if you're sensitive to any of the ingredients*

YIELDS: 1 reusable dryer sheet

➤ 1 (5" × 5") piece of cotton fabric (cut from an old 100 percent cotton T-shirt, undershirt, or other item that you'd like to repurpose)

➤ 2 drops essential oil of your choice

Apply essential oil to the cotton fabric before adding to the dryer.

remedy notes

These dryer sheets smell wonderful, but they don't prevent static cling. To prevent static while using natural dryer sheets, try adding dryer balls or tennis balls to the dryer to reduce friction between your clothes as they dry. Drying synthetic fibers in a separate load can help too. Also, do not use more than 2 drops of essential oil per sheet. Using too much oil could stain your clothing or even pose a fire risk.

Chapter 4

HAIR, SKIN, AND NAILS

Together, your hair, skin, and nails make up your integumentary system. This system's job is to protect your body from the elements, regulate your temperature, and convey a constant stream of sensory information to your nervous system. The recipes in this chapter will help keep your hair, skin, and nails looking and feeling their best.

The strength and beauty of your hair, skin, and nails reflect your overall well-being. Health comes from within, not just from what you apply topically. While you're enjoying beautifying recipes like the Luxurious Toner for All Skin Types and the Coconut Citrus Cuticle Treatment found in this chapter, remember to drink nourishing Stinging Nettle Infusion for Strong Hair, Nails, and Teeth a few times per week to keep these parts of your body strong and gorgeous.

Stress, hormonal fluctuations, blood sugar issues, dehydration, and lack of exercise can all set the stage for skin woes or weakened hair and nails. That's why you'll get the best results if you combine the recipes in this chapter with remedies from later chapters that can help to address the root of the problem. Check out Chapter 7 for remedies to relieve stress, Chapter 9 for remedies to support detoxification through your liver and large intestine, and Chapter 10 for help with hormone balance.

✦ Customized Jojoba Facial Cleanser ✦

BENEFITS AND USES: *cleans your face and helps nourish your skin*

AVOID: *giving up on this oil before your skin adjusts*

YIELDS: 1 ounce (approximately 40 applications)

FOR ACNE-PRONE SKIN:
- 2 drops tea tree essential oil
- 5 drops German chamomile essential oil
- 3 drops rosemary essential oil

FOR SENSITIVE SKIN:
- 6 drops German chamomile essential oil

FOR DRY, DULL SKIN:
- 2 drops rosemary essential oil
- 2 drops geranium essential oil
- 2 drops lavender essential oil
- 2 drops German chamomile essential oil

FOR ALL OPTIONS:
- 2 tablespoons jojoba oil, divided

1 *To make the cleanser:* Add the essential oil blend of your choice to the bottom of a clean glass bottle. (A 1-ounce bottle with a dropper attached to the lid is ideal since 2 tablespoons of jojoba oil is equivalent to 1 ounce.) Then add 1 ounce jojoba oil before securing the lid and shaking to mix. Add the remaining 1 ounce jojoba oil and shake again.

Customized Jojoba Facial Cleanser—continued

2 *To use the cleanser:* Squirt ½ dropperful of the cleanser onto clean hands. Using small upward circular motions, massage the cleanser onto a dry face. (Important: apply the cleanser to dry skin! If you moisten your face first, it will have a harder time "adhering" to the makeup and dirt that's mixed with your sebum and this method won't be as effective.) After massaging the cleanser into your face for 1–5 minutes, use a warm, wet washcloth to remove the cleanser (and dirt and makeup!) from your face.

Soaps and foaming cleansers strip the natural oils from your skin, which can trigger breakouts, dryness, sensitivity, and even oiliness. This oil-based cleanser removes built-up grime without disrupting your skin's balance or clogging your pores. It's counterintuitive, but oily skin becomes less oily once it's not trying to overcompensate. When you start using this cleansing method, it might take a few weeks for your skin to rebalance. The results are worth the wait.

⊁ Activated Charcoal ⊁
Acne Spot Treatment

BENEFITS AND USES: *helps with painful, cystic acne that erupts on otherwise normal to oily skin*

AVOID: *if your skin is very dry*

YIELDS: 1 treatment

- 1 (500-milligram) activated charcoal capsule
- ⅛ cup fresh aloe vera gel (see Aloe Vera recipe in Chapter 3)
- 2 drops tea tree essential oil

1 Open the capsule of activated charcoal by pulling or twisting the two pieces of the capsule apart over a small bowl. Once the capsule is opened, empty the contents into the bowl.

2 Add aloe gel to the bowl. Using a fork, mash the aloe into the charcoal until the two are roughly combined, about 60 seconds.

3 Add tea tree essential oil and mix until everything seems evenly distributed, about another 15 seconds.

4 Use your fingers to apply the mixture to clean, dry skin. Cover any pimples and include about 1 inch of skin around each blemish. Avoid getting this mixture in your eyes or on the delicate skin underneath your eyes.

5 Leave on at least 20 minutes. Wipe off with a clean towel or washcloth dampened with warm water.

remedy notes

Cystic acne is often triggered by hormonal fluctuations, but this treatment can help to lessen the size, redness, and severity of a blemish once it erupts. Try the Dandelion Root Liver Cleanse (see Chapter 9) to help prevent cystic acne from forming.

Lavender Honey Mask

BENEFITS AND USES: *prevents and treats small pimples accompanied by dryness and irritation*

AVOID: *if you're allergic to lavender or honey*

YIELDS: 1 treatment

> **1 tablespoon raw honey**
> **3 drops lavender essential oil**

1 Put honey in a small, clean bowl.

2 Add lavender essential oil and stir to combine.

3 Using clean fingertips, apply the mask to the entire face except the eye area. Avoid your hairline unless you're taking a shower right after the treatment to avoid getting any honey in your hair.

4 Leave on at least 20 minutes or up to 2 hours. This treatment isn't ideal for overnight use or for use during a hot bath. The honey can get messy! Remove with a clean washcloth and warm water.

remedy notes

Lavender and honey are gentle ingredients that both have antimicrobial properties and support skin healing, which makes this soothing treatment the best remedy for acne that erupts on sensitive or dry skin. You can also use it as a moisturizing treatment whether or not you have acne. If you don't want to apply this treatment as a face mask, just dab a small amount of honey and a drop of lavender essential oil on a small area as an acne spot treatment.

⤜ Luxurious Toner for All Skin Types ⤛

BENEFITS AND USES: *helps with all-around pampering of your skin!*

AVOID: *if your skin feels "tight" after using*

YIELDS: about 1 quart

FOR ALL RECIPE OPTIONS:

▸ ¼ cup dried lavender flowers

▸ ¼ cup dried chamomile flowers

▸ ¼ cup dried rose petals

▸ ¼ cup dried calendula flowers, packed

▸ ¼ cup chopped fresh plantain leaf (see Chapter 2)

▸ 1 tablespoon organic lemon zest

▸ 1 tablespoon dried rosemary (or 2 sprigs fresh rosemary)

▸ 1 tablespoon dried sage (or 2 sprigs fresh sage)

▸ 3 cups apple cider vinegar

▸ 2 cups rose water

FOR ACNE-PRONE SKIN:

▸ 5 drops rosemary essential oil

▸ 5 drops lavender essential oil

▸ 2 drops tea tree essential oil

▸ 7 drops German chamomile essential oil

FOR SENSITIVE SKIN OR SKIN THAT'S PRONE TO REDNESS:

▸ 10 drops German chamomile essential oil

FOR ROSACEA AND/OR BROKEN CAPILLARIES:

▸ 8 drops geranium essential oil

▸ 8 drops German chamomile essential oil

Luxurious Toner for All Skin Types—continued

1 Add lavender, chamomile, rose petals, calendula flowers, plantain, lemon zest, rosemary, and sage to a quart-sized glass Mason jar. Cover herb mixture with apple cider vinegar. Cover with a plastic lid and shake until herbs are saturated.

2 Let herbs steep in vinegar for at least 2 weeks and up to 4 weeks, until the vinegar takes on a complex herbal fragrance. In warmer weather, 2 weeks might be enough time. If it's chilly in your house, wait a little longer. Shake the jar a few times per week. If the herbs absorb enough of the vinegar so that they aren't staying covered, add more vinegar.

3 Once herbs are done steeping, strain liquid using a fine-mesh sieve lined with cheesecloth or an unbleached paper towel. Squeeze the spent herbs to extract as much vinegar as possible.

4 After straining, you should have about 2 cups infused vinegar. Dilute with an equal amount of rose water. Then add essential oils, replace the lid, and shake vigorously to combine.

5 To use, simply dab onto clean skin and gently pat with clean hands until absorbed. If you prefer, store the toner in a spray bottle and spray it onto your skin for a hands-free application.

remedy notes

Healthy skin is protected by an acid mantle, so products like this one that are slightly acidic are a great match for your skin's natural barrier. Here, lavender and chamomile help to heal blemishes, rose helps to calm inflammation and offers protective antioxidants, and calendula and plantain encourage skin repair. The apple cider vinegar is more than just a vehicle for all the benefits of the herbs; it helps the final formula to achieve the perfect pH. Avoid using any essential oils that are already diluted in a carrier oil; since oil and water don't mix, a pre-diluted essential oil won't dissolve into the formula.

Antioxidant and Tea Tree Toner for Oily Skin

BENEFITS AND USES: *helps your skin balance its oil production without causing dryness*

AVOID: *if your skin feels "tight" after using*

YIELDS: about 1½ cups

- ¼ cup dried calendula flowers, tightly packed
- ⅛ cup dried green tea leaves
- ⅛ cup rose hips
- 1 cup alcohol-free witch hazel distillate
- ¼ cup apple cider vinegar
- 1 cup rose water
- 5 drops tea tree essential oil

---

1 Add calendula flowers, green tea leaves, and rose hips to a Mason jar. Cover with witch hazel distillate and apple cider vinegar. Screw cover onto jar and shake well. Allow this mixture to steep at least 2 weeks and up to 4 weeks. Shake the jar a few times per week. You'll know it's ready when the color of the liquid changes slightly.

2 Strain the herbs from the liquid. Add rose water and tea tree essential oil. Screw cover onto jar and shake well to combine.

3 To use the toner, shake well before using and dab onto clean skin with a cotton ball or clean hands. Avoid contact with eyes and the delicate skin surrounding them. You can also store it in a fine mist spritz bottle and spray it onto your skin (while your eyes are closed!) instead.

⋙ Oat and Almond Body Scrub ⋘

BENEFITS AND USES: *softens and exfoliates normal to dry skin*

AVOID: *using on your face or on broken skin*

YIELDS: about ½ cup

- ¼ **cup raw unsalted almonds**
- ¼ **cup rolled oats**
- **1 tablespoon dried rose petals**
- **1 tablespoon dried lavender flowers**
- ¾ **cup extra-virgin olive oil**

1 Measure almonds and oats into a food processor. Pulse 5 seconds at a time until the mixture looks like fine sand, about 1½ minutes.

2 Add rose petals and lavender flowers. Pulse three times for 1–2 seconds each until petals are roughly chopped and distributed throughout the mixture. This dry mixture will keep 3–4 weeks in a cool, dry cupboard. You can make a double or quadruple batch in advance and store it in a zip-top "freezer" bag, Tupperware-style container, or Mason jar for future use.

3 When you're ready to use the treatment, saturate the mixture with olive oil and stir to combine. Using clean fingers, massage generously and vigorously into damp skin, using upward, circular motions. Always direct your strokes from the periphery of your body toward your heart. For best results, use this scrub at least twice per week. Do not exceed one use per day.

4 Rinse off with warm water and enjoy how soft and smooth your skin is! Make sure to use a stopper in the drain so that the oats and almonds don't clog your plumbing.

5 Once you've added the olive oil, store any leftover scrub in a covered container in the fridge no longer than 1 week.

✈ Peppermint White Chocolate Body Butter ✈

YIELDS: 2 cups

- ½ cup cocoa butter
- ¼ cup plus 1 tablespoon unrefined coconut oil
- ¼ cup plus 1 tablespoon jojoba oil
- 1 tablespoon arrowroot powder
- 20 drops peppermint essential oil

1 Set up a double boiler by filling a small pot with 2"–3" of hot water and situating a heat-safe glass bowl atop the pot. Be sure that the glass is not touching the water. Apply moderate heat so that the water comes to a simmer and add the cocoa butter to the glass bowl. Use this method to melt the cocoa butter very slowly over low heat, stirring as needed to encourage even melting. As soon as the cocoa butter is melted, turn off the heat, leaving the glass bowl in place.

2 Add the coconut oil and jojoba oil to the glass bowl, stirring vigorously so that the coconut oil melts completely and the oils and butter are well mixed. Remove the glass bowl from the pot (use potholders!) and whisk in the arrowroot powder and peppermint essential oil until the mixture is smooth.

3 Place the mixture in the fridge 1–2 hours, or in the freezer 15–20 minutes. Remove when texture appears slightly creamy but is still malleable enough to scoop up with a spoon.

4 Using a hand mixer or a stand mixer, whip the mixture on low speed for 30 seconds and slowly increase the speed to high. Continue whipping on high speed until it doubles in size and looks like whipped frosting, about 6–8 minutes.

5 To use, simply massage into your skin. Store in a covered container with a wide opening (such as a tin or plastic tub) at cool room temperature up to 2 months. If the butter melts, repeat steps 3 and 4 to re-whip it before using.

✈ Soothing Oat and Calendula Bath ✈

BENEFITS AND USES: *soothes itchy, dry, and/or inflamed skin*

AVOID: *using overly hot water in the bath, which can further irritate the skin*

YIELDS: 1 treatment

- ½ cup rolled oats
- ¼ cup dried calendula flowers
- 3 drops German chamomile essential oil
- 2 drops lavender essential oil
- A nylon stocking, trouser sock, or long sock made of thin cotton

1 Combine all ingredients except stocking in a clean bowl. Stir to combine.

2 Fill the stocking with the oat and flower mixture and then tie a knot at the top to keep the stocking closed.

3 Place the stuffed stocking into the tub and draw a warm bath.

4 Soak in the medicinal bath for 20–30 minutes. You can use the stocking like a bath sponge. Gently squeeze it under the water and over the skin to release the soothing properties of the mixture into the bathwater and directly onto the skin.

5 Discard stocking after use and rinse tub thoroughly to remove any residue.

 remedy notes

This is a gentle way to soothe eczema and psoriasis, or to bring relief to the itching that comes with chicken pox. You can also use this as a gentle moisturizing bath for all skin types.

☞ Coconut Oil Body Balm ☜

BENEFITS AND USES: *moisturizes and protects your skin*

AVOID: *using on your face and/or genitals*

YIELDS: about 1½ cups

- 1½ cups virgin coconut oil
- 2½ tablespoons coarsely ground coffee beans
- ¼ cup jojoba oil
- 2 tablespoons shaved or pelleted beeswax
- 5 drops nutmeg essential oil

1 Place coconut oil and ground coffee in a small pot and heat on low. Once the oil is completely liquefied, about 2–3 minutes, turn off the heat. Let stand at least 2 hours to allow the coffee to infuse. If it's cold in your kitchen, check the pot periodically to make sure that the oil stays liquid while infusing. If the oil starts to solidify, turn on the heat for a few minutes.

2 Once the coconut oil has infused, strain it through a fine-mesh sieve lined with cheesecloth to remove all of the coffee particles.

3 Wipe out the pot with paper towels until no coffee grounds remain. Return the infused coconut oil to the pot and add jojoba oil and beeswax. Turn the heat on low and stir continuously until beeswax is completely melted. Once wax is melted, turn off heat.

4 *For a solid body balm:* Add the nutmeg essential oil and stir once to combine before pouring into containers. Small metal tins made for salves are ideal for this balm, and this recipe will fill four 4-ounce tins. If you don't want to purchase tins, you can use a small plastic food storage container with a lid—just make sure to wait until the balm is cool enough to touch before pouring into plastic.

Coconut Oil Body Balm—continued

5 *For a whipped body balm:* Pour the wax mixture into the bowl of your stand mixer and refrigerate until cool to the touch and slightly creamy in appearance, about 1–2 hours. Once cool, whip on low speed for 30 seconds, then slowly increase the speed to high and continue whipping about 8 minutes or until the balm becomes billowy and soft, almost doubling in volume. Add nutmeg essential oil and whip on low speed 1 additional minute to distribute. Use a spatula to dispense into tins or small wide-mouth Mason jars and store at cool room temperature up to 2 months.

6 To use the balm, simply apply with clean fingers to any part of your body (except your face and genitals) to moisturize.

remedy notes

Skin is a semipermeable membrane that breathes, eliminates waste products, and plays a role in helping your body to detoxify itself. This semipermeable nature is the reason why skin eagerly absorbs many of the ingredients in the products that you use. Using food-grade ingredients, like all of the recipes in this chapter do, is one way to ensure that your skin isn't soaking up anything from your skincare regimen that doesn't belong in your body.

⇥ Stinging Nettle Infusion ⇤
for Strong Hair, Nails, and Teeth

BENEFITS AND USES: *strengthens and beautifies your body from the inside out*

AVOID: *combining with blood thinners that require you to be careful about vitamin K levels. If you have any doubts, ask your prescribing physician.*

YIELDS: 2 servings

▸ **1 heaping cup dried stinging nettle leaf**

▸ **Scant 4 cups water**

1 Place stinging nettle leaf at the bottom of a quart-sized Mason jar.

2 Boil water and pour it over the stinging nettle leaf in the jar.

3 Stir stinging nettle leaf so that it is fully saturated with hot water and then let the mixture steep on the counter at least 4 hours or overnight.

4 When you're ready to drink the infusion, strain it through cheesecloth, a nut milk bag, or a fine-mesh sieve and drink. You can reheat it if desired, or serve it chilled. Store any leftovers in the fridge and drink within 24 hours.

remedy notes

This rich infusion supports healthy hair, nails, teeth, and bones by providing your body with easy-to-absorb vitamins and minerals, including magnesium, calcium, iron, potassium, and vitamins A, C, and K. Enjoy this infusion a few times per week for maintenance or, if you're struggling with weak hair, splitting nails, osteopenia, anemia, or fatigue, drink at least one serving per day until your condition improves. If you don't like the taste of the infusion at first, try substituting half of the nettle leaf with peppermint leaves or stirring in some miso paste to create a savory "broth."

Coconut Citrus Cuticle Treatment

BENEFITS AND USES: *softens cuticles and nourishes nail beds*

AVOID: *if you're allergic to citrus or coconut*

YIELDS: 1 treatment

> ½ tablespoon organic citrus zest of your choice (lemon, lime, orange—whatever you have on hand)

> 1 tablespoon coconut oil

---

1 Mix citrus zest with coconut oil in a small, microwave-safe bowl.

2 Microwave on high for 15 seconds. Remove from microwave and stir, checking to see if the oil is liquefied and just barely warm. If oil isn't warmed all the way through, return to the microwave another 10 seconds and stir again. Once oil is warm, the treatment is ready to use.

3 To apply treatment, use small, circular motions to gently massage oil into your nails and cuticles. Then use your fingers or a cuticle-pusher tool to gently push down your cuticles. (Don't forget your toes!)

4 After 30 minutes, wipe away the excess oil and remaining citrus zest with a clean towel.

remedy notes

If you're going to continue with a manicure right after this treatment, you might want to wipe your nail beds with nail polish remover to be sure that you've removed every last trace of oil. Otherwise, your nail polish might not adhere.

⤛ Warm Oil Hair Treatment ⤜

BENEFITS AND USES: *imparts deep moisture to normal to dry hair*

AVOID: *using right before a big day since your hair may feel heavy for a day or two after use*

YIELDS: 1 cup

> ▸ **1 cup jojoba oil**

1 Gently warm oil in a small pot over low heat about 5 minutes or until oil is pleasantly warm to the touch, not hot. Do not leave oil unattended or allow it to overheat!

2 Using your fingertips, massage about 1½ tablespoons warm oil into your roots to stimulate circulation and exfoliate your scalp.

3 Spend at least 3 minutes massaging the oil into your scalp. If you have more time, spend up to 10 minutes on this step. When you're finished massaging, apply the remainder of the oil generously to the ends and length of the hair. If you have short hair, you might need only another tablespoon or two. If you have waist-length hair, you may need the whole cup of oil to fully saturate the strands. *Note: the more hair you have, the more oil you'll need to fully saturate your hair.*

4 Secure your hair under a plastic bag or shower cap. If your hair is long, you might like to braid it so that it stays together more comfortably under the plastic. The plastic will hold the heat and allow the oil to penetrate your hair for best results.

5 Leave on at least 20 minutes and up to overnight.

Warm Oil Hair Treatment—continued

6   When you're ready to remove the oil, squeeze as much oil from your hair as you can with a clean towel. (Keep in mind that oil may stain the towel, so choose an old towel for this task.) Apply shampoo directly to the treated hair without adding water first and work into a lather for 3 minutes before adding water. Shampoo thoroughly, rinse hair, and shampoo again. Apply conditioner and dry your hair as you normally would. If your hair is fine, it might take another day or two of regular shampooing to fully remove the heaviness of the oil.

7   For normal hair, repeat this treatment two to three times per month. For dry hair, repeat as often as three times per week until your hair's condition improves.

You can customize this treatment by using olive oil instead of jojoba and/or by adding essential oils for fragrance or for their specific properties. For dandruff, try adding 20 drops rosemary and 20 drops clary sage. Try 15 drops German chamomile with 25 drops lavender for redness and irritation, or 25 drops lavender and 10 drops tea tree if you're prone to acne near your hairline.

⁕ Rosemary and Geranium Scalp Oil ⁕

BENEFITS AND USES: *encourages hair growth and balanced oil production*

AVOID: *using while pregnant*

YIELDS: about 30 applications

> **20 drops rosemary essential oil**
> **15 drops geranium essential oil**
> **2 tablespoons jojoba oil, divided**

1 Add the essential oils to the bottom of a clean glass bottle. (A 1-ounce bottle with a dropper attached to the lid is ideal.) Add 1 tablespoon jojoba oil, secure the lid, and shake to mix. Add remaining 1 tablespoon jojoba oil, secure the lid, and shake again. Label the bottle and store away from extreme temperatures and bright light until ready to use.

2 To use, dispense 1 dropperful onto clean fingertips and massage vigorously into the scalp. Use more oil as needed to ensure that all of your scalp receives some of the treatment. Leave the oil on at least 20 minutes (it's okay to leave it on up to an hour or two, if your time allows), then shampoo and condition as normal. For best results, apply the treatment three times per week.

remedy notes

When thinning hair is the result of stress, poor circulation, or nutrient depletion, natural remedies can make a big difference. Applying this oil as directed, in combination with drinking Stinging Nettle Infusion for Strong Hair, Nails, and Teeth (see recipe in this chapter) every day, can slow or stop hair loss in 2–3 weeks and strengthen hair when it regrows.

⤜ Apple Cider Vinegar ⤛
Anti-Dandruff Rinse

BENEFITS AND USES: *helps with mild to moderate dandruff*

AVOID: *if you have dry hair, eczema, or psoriasis, or if the vinegar causes scalp discomfort*

YIELDS: 4 treatments

- **1 cup apple cider vinegar**
- **20 drops clary sage essential oil**
- **20 drops lavender essential oil**
- **1 cup water, divided**

1 Add apple cider vinegar and essential oils to a quart-sized glass jar and stir well to combine. (Mason jars work well, but use a plastic lid. Vinegar can erode the standard rubber and metal lids.) Label the jar, including the date and ingredients along with instructions to dilute with an equal volume of water before using. Store at room temperature away from bright light up to 1 year, but use within 3 months for best results.

2 When you're ready to use the treatment, measure out ¼ cup into a plastic container that's safe to take into the shower or bath. Add ¼ cup water to make one treatment.

3 Before shampooing your hair, pour the treatment generously over your scalp and roots. Massage it into your hair thoroughly, then shampoo and condition as normal.

4 Repeat one to two times per week until the scalp isn't flaking anymore.

remedy notes

If your hair and scalp are dry, alternate this treatment with the Warm Oil Hair Treatment (see recipe in this chapter) to prevent this rinse from drying out your hair too much. Use each treatment at least once per week.

❧ Rosemary Hair Rinse ❧

YIELDS: 4 treatments

> 1¼ cups apple cider vinegar
> ¼ cup fresh rosemary sprigs, loosely packed
> 10 drops rosemary essential oil
> 10 drops lavender essential oil
> 1 cup water, divided

1 Add apple cider vinegar and rosemary sprigs to a small, heavy-bottomed pot and partially cover with a lid. Apply moderate heat until vinegar barely starts to come to a simmer and allow to simmer gently for 5 minutes. After 5 minutes, secure the lid and turn off the heat. Let stand on the same burner, fully covered, at least 30 minutes.

2 Strain infused vinegar through a small fine-mesh sieve into a quart-sized jar or container. Discard rosemary sprigs. Add essential oils and stir to combine. If you won't be using the treatment right away, store in a glass jar or plastic container with a label that says, "Do not drink." If you keep the labeled jar away from extreme temperatures and bright light, it will maintain peak potency for 3 months but will still be safe to use for up to 1 year.

3 To use the treatment, stir or shake container to distribute any essential oils, then measure out ¼ cup infused vinegar into a plastic bowl (it's best to avoid bringing glass into the shower or bath). Add ¼ cup water to make one treatment.

Rosemary Hair Rinse—continued

4 Bring the treatment with you to the shower or bath, wet your hair and scalp with warm water, and pour the rinse over your scalp and roots. Most of the liquid will seem to run right over your hair, but don't worry—this quick rinse is plenty. Massage your hair and scalp to help it soak in, then shampoo and condition your hair as normal.

5 For normal hair, repeat this up to twice per month. If your hair is oily or flaky, or if you have a lot of buildup from hair products, use this treatment as frequently as twice per week.

remedy notes

This hair rinse is a quick way to restore shine and body to your hair. The apple cider vinegar helps to clear away residue that builds up over time as you shampoo, condition, and style your hair. Rosemary encourages hair growth and fights dandruff, while lavender soothes your scalp and balances oil production.

Emergency Cayenne Pepper "Band-Aid"

BENEFITS AND USES: *helps with small cuts*

AVOID: *if the edges of the cut don't meet*

YIELDS: 1 treatment

▸ **1 teaspoon cayenne pepper**

1 Place cayenne pepper on a small plate.

2 Wash the cut with soap and water to disinfect. Pat dry with a clean towel.

3 Press the cut into the pile of cayenne pepper.

4 Use a clean towel to apply continuous pressure to the cayenne-covered cut until the bleeding has completely stopped. *Note: if this takes longer than 2 minutes, you might need to call a doctor or head to urgent care or the ER for stitches.* Cover with a bandage, leaving the cayenne pepper in place until it flakes off on its own. Discard any cayenne pepper remaining on the plate.

remedy notes

Cayenne helps your body to form an effective clot to stop bleeding quickly. It also has antimicrobial properties and can relieve pain. Don't touch your eyes, nose, mouth, or genitals after using this remedy until the cayenne is covered securely with a bandage and you've washed your hands.

⤞ Fresh Plantain Leaf ⤝ for Cuts and Scrapes

BENEFITS AND USES: *soothes minor cuts, bumps, scratches, and bug bites when playing outside*

AVOID: *using plantain on a puncture wound*

YIELDS: 1 treatment

▸ **3–6 fresh plantain leaves (3 broad leaves or 6 skinny ones)**

Dust off the leaves as best you can or rinse them in a water fountain, if available. Chew the leaves for 30 seconds to crush them and apply the chewed plant matter directly to the affected area. Hold in place for at least 5 minutes or until you can clean the wound and apply a bandage.

remedy notes

Plantain can be a great help when you don't have access to a first aid kit. Some herbalists refer to it as "playground medicine" because it's so helpful for soothing the minor "boo-boos" kids tend to get while playing outside. Also, plantain tends to grow in tightly packed ground where there's been a lot of foot traffic; playgrounds are a perfect example of its favorite habitat. Part of plantain's magic is that it's usually no more than a few feet away when you need it.

First Aid Salve
with Yarrow, Calendula, and Plantain

BENEFITS AND USES: *tends to cuts, scrapes, abrasions, and bruises. All of the herbs in this formula are powerful wound-healing herbs. When combined in this salve, they help cuts, scrapes, and bruises to heal more quickly and completely.*

AVOID: *if the wound is infected or needs stitches, or if it's a puncture wound. Never use salve of any kind on a puncture wound!*

YIELDS: 8 (1-ounce) tins

- ½ cup fresh plantain leaves
- ¼ cup dried calendula flowers
- ¼ cup dried yarrow
- 1 cup extra-virgin olive oil
- 2 tablespoons shaved or pelleted beeswax
- 8 drops rosemary essential oil, divided
- 8 drops German chamomile essential oil, divided
- 8 drops lavender essential oil, divided
- 8 (1-ounce capacity) metal tins or jars to hold the finished salve

1 Spread out plantain leaves in a single layer on a clean towel and leave out to wilt for 12–24 hours.

2 Combine wilted plantain leaves, dried calendula flowers, and yarrow with olive oil in a double boiler. Warm over very low heat for about 2 hours without letting the temperature rise above 120°F. If you don't have a candy thermometer, the best way to do this is to alternate 20 minutes "on" (applying low heat to the double boiler) with 20–30 minutes "off" (letting the mixture stand on the burner with the heat off). After infusing, the oil will have a greenish hue and a faint herbal scent.

First Aid Salve with Yarrow, Calendula, and Plantain—continued

3 While the oil is still warm, strain the mixture through a fine-mesh sieve or a triple layer of cheesecloth into a clean pint- or quart-sized Mason jar. Add the beeswax directly to the warm oil and stir to dissolve, about 2–3 minutes depending on the size of the beeswax pieces. If the beeswax does not liquefy after 3 minutes of stirring, gently rewarm the contents of the jar by submerging it in a hot water bath and stir until wax has melted.

4 Open the tins and set them up in a row next to one another to make these final steps as easy and neat as possible. Place 1 drop of each essential oil into each empty tin.

5 Once essential oils have been added, immediately pour the liquefied oil and wax mixture into the tins. Divide the oil evenly between all eight tins, pouring approximately 1½ tablespoons into each. Set aside and cool to room temperature, then place lids on top. Store finished salve away from extreme temperatures for up to 2 years.

6 Apply the salve to cuts, scrapes, bruises, bug bites, chapped lips, and other minor skin irritations.

remedy notes

If you have an electric yogurt maker or a dehydrator, you could use one of these to provide gentle heat instead of the double boiler method. No matter what method you choose, it's very important not to let the temperature get too high. You're not trying to make fried herbs!

Baking Soda and Lavender Paste
for Bites and Stings

BENEFITS AND USES: *soothes bug bites and stings right after they happen*

AVOID: *if you experience rapid swelling, anaphylaxis, fever, or difficulty breathing*

YIELDS: 1 treatment

› **2 teaspoons baking soda**
› **25 drops lavender essential oil**

1 Place baking soda in a clean dish, then saturate with lavender essential oil. Stir, if needed, to make a paste.

2 Apply to the site of the bug bite until the affected area is completely covered.

3 Leave on 20–30 minutes. Remove with a cool, damp washcloth using a dabbing motion to avoid irritating the bug bite and reactivating the itchy sensation through friction.

remedy notes

This is a great remedy for both adults and children. The baking soda relieves irritation, and the lavender not only helps to soothe the affected skin, but it also helps children release some of the emotional upset that comes with a bad bug bite or bee sting. Keep in mind that you can make and apply more paste as needed. If you notice lots of heat or swelling or an unusual rash appearing around the site, consult a medical professional.

Aloe Vera Gel with Lavender and German Chamomile

BENEFITS AND USES: *speeds the healing process for minor burns, regenerates skin, and restores moisture*

AVOID: *if you have a serious wound*

YIELDS: about 1 ounce

> 2 tablespoons fresh aloe vera gel (see Aloe Vera recipe in Chapter 3)
> 5 drops lavender essential oil
> 3 drops German chamomile essential oil
> 1 drop rosemary essential oil

1 In a blender or food processor combine all ingredients. Blend on high until smooth, about 30–45 seconds.

2 *To speed the healing of minor burns:* Apply a generous layer to the affected areas three times per day. If you cover the area with a bandage to protect the skin, make sure to use a bandage that allows the skin to "breathe."

3 *To use as a hydrating facial mask:* After cleansing your skin (use the Customized Jojoba Facial Cleanser in this chapter for best results), lie on your back and apply a thick layer of this gel to your face. Leave on for 20 minutes before removing with a warm, damp washcloth. Follow with a few drops of jojoba oil or your favorite facial moisturizer.

4 Store leftovers in a clean glass jar in the refrigerator up to 1 week. If the gel begins to discolor, separate, or have an "off" odor, throw it away and make a new batch.

 remedy notes Always use a clean utensil to dispense skincare products. Avoid putting your fingers directly into the jar, as this will cause bacterial contamination and could reduce the shelf life of your remedies.

Black Tea and Lavender Sunburn Compress

BENEFITS AND USES: *relieves the pain of first- and second-degree sunburns*

AVOID: *if blisters cover more than 20 percent of your body or if you're experiencing dizziness, nausea, vomiting, fever, or chills after a sunburn*

YIELDS: 1 treatment

- 3 cups room temperature water, divided
- 4 black tea bags
- 1 cup ice
- 10 drops lavender essential oil

1 Boil 2 cups water.

2 Place tea bags in a large heat-safe tub or bowl. Pour boiling water over tea bags and let steep 15 minutes or until the water has turned a deep chestnut brown.

3 Remove tea bags, making sure to squeeze out as much liquid from them as possible before discarding. Add ice and stir until dissolved and then stir in remaining 1 cup water and lavender essential oil.

4 Saturate a clean washcloth or hand towel with tea mixture. (Use an old or dark-colored washcloth that you don't mind staining.) Squeeze out excess so that the compress is heavy with liquid but not dripping. Place prepared compress in a separate bowl and store any extra tea mixture in the fridge before taking the compress to a comfortable spot where you can rest.

5 Place compress over affected area. When the side of the compress that's against the skin begins to feel warm, flip the compress to the other side. Avoid rubbing the burned skin with the compress, and be careful not to drip since black tea can stain fabric and furniture.

Black Tea and Lavender Sunburn Compress—continued

6 When the entire compress feels warm (usually after 10–15 minutes), you can end the treatment or refresh the compress by returning it to the chilled tea and repeating the application. Discard any leftover tea that's been in direct contact with the compress. Tea that hasn't been in direct contact with the compress can be stored in the fridge overnight and used the following day, if needed.

remedy notes

The tannins in black tea act instantly to astringe weepy skin and relieve swelling. Lavender essential oil helps to speed the skin's healing process. This remedy relieves the pain of sunburn but doesn't undo the UV damage that increases your risk for skin cancer. Avoiding sunburn in the first place is the best policy!

⇥ Calendula Honey Lip Treatment ⇤

BENEFITS AND USES: *heals and moisturizes dry, chapped lips*

AVOID: *licking the honey off your lips*

YIELDS: about ½ cup
> 1 tablespoon dried calendula flowers
> ½ cup raw honey

1 Place calendula flowers in the bottom of a clean pint-sized glass jar.

2 Set up a double boiler by filling a small pot with 2"–3" of hot water and situating a heat-safe glass bowl atop the pot. Be sure that the glass is not touching the water. Turn on the burner to moderate heat to bring the water in the pot up to a simmer, then reduce heat to low and add the honey to the glass bowl. Gently warm the honey until it's warm to the touch but not too hot to handle, about 5–8 minutes. Avoid overheating the honey, as this compromises some of its medicinal properties.

3 Pour the warm honey over the calendula flowers and stir gently with a knife to make sure the flowers are completely submerged and coated by the honey.

4 Place jar in a warm spot (a sunny windowsill is a great choice) and allow the honey to infuse at least 5 days and up to 1 month, until it has a mild floral note when you taste a drop of it. When the infusion is complete, strain the honey through a fine-mesh sieve into a clean jar. (If you're having trouble straining it, you can warm the mixture using a double boiler as you did in step 1 to make it easier to pour through the sieve.) Store in a covered jar at cool room temperature up to 1 year.

5 To use, pour a small amount onto your finger and apply directly to clean lips. Avoid dipping your fingers into the honey jar, as this can cause contamination. For best results, use this treatment once or twice daily and avoid using lip balms with petroleum-based ingredients or menthol.

Chapter 5

IMMUNE AND RESPIRATORY SYSTEMS

Traditional Chinese Medicine pictures the body's self-protective force as an energy that dwells in the pores of the skin. The teachings tell us that this wei qi, or protective energy, is governed by the Lung and Large Intestine meridians and will become stronger with appropriate nourishment, breathing, and exercise but will be weakened by grief. As remote as some of these traditional ideas might seem from modern understandings of the immune and respiratory systems, they do overlap with modern discoveries about the roles that nutrition, gut health, and emotional balance play in determining how well our immune systems function.

In this chapter you'll find recipes supported by modern scientific understanding of the immune system and traditional wisdom alike. You'll learn how to keep your immune system balanced with nourishing recipes that support gut flora through their probiotic content (Lacto-Fermented Sauerkraut and multiple recipes using miso paste) and how to make delicious soups that deliver traditional immune system tonics like astragalus (Immune-Boosting Broth with Shiitake and Astragalus). You'll make your own versions of some of herbal medicine's "greatest hits," including a sweet Elderberry Spice Syrup and spicy Classic Fire Cider. And if your efforts at prevention aren't quite enough to keep that cold, flu, or sinus infection at bay, this chapter will show you how to take care of yourself so that your recovery will be as quick and easy as possible.

⤞ Grapefruit and Tea Tree ⤝ Foaming Hand Soap

BENEFITS AND USES: *helps you stay healthy during cold and flu season*

AVOID: *contact with eyes*

YIELDS: 8 ounces

- ⅞ **cup water**
- ½ **teaspoon jojoba oil**
- **2 tablespoons liquid castile soap**
- **10 drops grapefruit essential oil**
- **5 drops tea tree essential oil**

1 Add all ingredients to a foaming soap dispenser. Shake or stir to combine.

2 To use: wet your hands with warm (not hot) water, dispense 1–2 pumps of this soap, and rub your hands together for as long as it takes to sing "Happy Birthday." Rinse with warm water.

remedy notes

Washing your hands after using the bathroom, before eating, and before food preparation is the single most important thing you can do to avoid getting sick. And the most important ingredient in this recipe is the friction you use when you wash your hands. It's the action of rubbing your hands together that does the most to get them clean.

Tea Tree and Rosemary Sinus Steam

BENEFITS AND USES: *opens up clogged sinuses and relieves upper respiratory infections*

AVOID: *creating a fire hazard by letting long hair, clothing, or a towel hang over the burner while it's still on*

YIELDS: 1 treatment

- **Water to cover**
- **7 drops tea tree essential oil**
- **7 drops rosemary essential oil**
- **1 bath towel**

1 Choose a pot or pan with a wide diameter. Add water until it's 2"–3" inches deep and warm over high heat.

2 Once the water reaches a rolling boil, turn off the heat. Wait a few seconds for the water to become still, then add essential oils to the water.

3 Bend over at the waist so that your head is about 15"–25" from the surface of the water. Drape the towel over the back of your head so that it forms a "tent" over the pot. The towel will help to trap the steam so that you can breathe in a high concentration of moisture, warmth, and essential oils.

4 Continue treatment for 10–15 minutes, taking as many breaks as you need. If your face feels too hot, if you're having any difficulty breathing, or if you feel light-headed, make sure to take a break. Repeat as often as desired.

remedy notes

When you blow your nose, check the color of the mucus for an important clue about what's happening in your sinuses. If the mucus is clear or white and you have symptoms like congestion and a runny nose, the most likely culprit is a virus. Green or yellow mucus is probably due to a bacterial and/or fungal infection. Fungal sinus infections are particularly hard to treat, but steaming the sinuses with tea tree essential oil twice per day can make a big difference.

⊹ Lacto-Fermented Sauerkraut ⊹

BENEFITS AND USES: *populates your digestive tract with beneficial bacteria (probiotics) to strengthen your immune system*

AVOID: *if you cannot tolerate cabbage; limit your intake if you're following a low-sodium diet*

YIELDS: 12 servings

- **1 head green cabbage, thinly sliced, divided**
- **3 teaspoons sea salt, divided**

1. Add a layer of cabbage to a large bowl and sprinkle with ¼ teaspoon sea salt. Cover with a second layer of cabbage and sprinkle another ¼ teaspoon salt over that layer too. Continue layering salt and cabbage until all of the cabbage has been added to the bowl. Make sure to end with a final layer of ¼ teaspoon salt.

2. With clean hands, massage the salt into the cabbage until all of the cabbage is soft and starts to release liquid—about 5 minutes of massaging with firm pressure should do the trick.

3. Pack the softened cabbage into a large, wide-mouthed, quart-sized Mason jar. (Depending on the size of your cabbage, you may need more than one jar to hold all of your sauerkraut!) Press the cabbage down so that it is completely covered by its liquid. Don't let any of the cabbage stick out into the air—this can cause the batch to spoil.

4. Find a small cup that will fit inside the mouth of the Mason jar and fill it with something heavy: beans, coins, clean stones, etc. Place the weighted cup inside the mouth of the Mason jar so that it presses down the cabbage and keeps it submerged beneath the brine.

Lacto-Fermented Sauerkraut—continued

5   Cover the top of the Mason jar loosely with a cloth and allow to sit at room temperature for about 2 weeks. Check the kraut every day or so to make sure that all of the cabbage is still submerged. Use a clean chopstick as needed to release air bubbles by inserting it into the jar and poking around to see if you hit any pockets of air created by the probiotics. After each air bubble check, press the cabbage down below the brine again to prevent spoilage.

6   After 2 weeks, or as soon as you like the way it tastes, your kraut is ready! Once you reach a flavor and consistency you love, store your sauerkraut in a covered container in the fridge for up to 6 months. Enjoy at least one serving daily to keep your immune system strong.

remedy notes

Sauerkraut contains both probiotics (living organisms) and prebiotics (soluble fiber), which help populate your gut with beneficial bacteria that can enhance your immunity. Sea salt or kosher salt is necessary for this recipe since iodized salt may interfere with the growth of the good bacteria.

Miso Noodle Soup

BENEFITS AND USES: *delivers nutrients, medicinal compounds, and hydration while you're sick*

AVOID: *N/A*

YIELDS: 4 servings

- 1 tablespoon unrefined sesame oil
- 6 garlic cloves, peeled and minced
- 1 large onion, peeled and diced
- ¼ cup peeled and sliced fresh ginger root
- 1 tablespoon fresh thyme (or 1 teaspoon dried)
- 1 tablespoon fresh rosemary (or 1 teaspoon dried)
- ½ teaspoon dried sage
- 4½ cups water, divided
- Scant ⅛ teaspoon cayenne pepper
- 1 (12-ounce) package silken tofu
- 4 ounces buckwheat soba noodles
- 4 tablespoons unpasteurized miso paste, divided
- ½ bunch green onions, sliced, divided

1 Warm sesame oil in a medium-sized pot over moderate heat for 1–2 minutes until fragrant. Add garlic, onion, and ginger and cook 5–6 minutes, stirring occasionally, until the onion is soft and translucent.

2 While garlic mixture is cooking, bundle thyme, rosemary, and sage into a piece of cheesecloth and tie securely to prevent stray rosemary needles from falling into the soup.

3 Add ½ cup water to the pot and stir vigorously with a wooden spoon. Use the spoon to nudge any browned bits from the bottom of the pot to release the flavor of any onions that caramelized.

Miso Noodle Soup—continued

4 Add the rest of the water, the cheesecloth-wrapped herbs, and dash of cayenne to the pot. Bring to a rolling boil and then immediately reduce heat to a low simmer and cook uncovered for 15 minutes.

5 Remove the cheesecloth bundle and store the broth in the fridge in a covered container up to 5 days until you're ready to serve.

6 To serve, cut tofu into ½" squares and bring the pot of broth to a gentle simmer. Add the tofu squares to the broth. (If using previously made broth from the fridge, reheat the broth in a pot on the stovetop before adding the tofu.) Simmer 2–3 minutes to warm the tofu.

7 Prepare soba noodles in a separate pot according to package directions and set aside.

8 Add 1 tablespoon miso paste to each serving bowl. Add one ladleful of broth to each bowl to help dissolve the miso. Use the back of a spoon to break up the miso paste until it has dissolved completely and the broth looks thick and creamy. Add ½ cup cooked noodles and 1 additional cup broth (with tofu squares) to the bowl. Top with green onions and serve.

remedy notes

When you're not fighting an active infection, try adding some astragalus root for additional immune support. If using tongue depressor–shaped slices, add 6 slices directly to the water along with the bundled herbs and remove the astragalus when you remove the herb bundle. If using smaller "cut and sifted" root pieces, bundle 2 tablespoons into the cheesecloth along with the thyme, rosemary, and sage.

Clary Sage and Grapefruit Air Purifier

BENEFITS AND USES: *purifies the air during or after a respiratory illness*

AVOID: *diffusing essential oils in a room shared by cats*

YIELDS: 1 treatment

- 1 essential oil diffuser
- Water per manufacturer's instructions
- 3 drops clary sage essential oil
- 1 drop rosemary essential oil
- 5 drops grapefruit essential oil

Fill your diffuser with water according to the manufacturer's instructions. Add essential oils and operate the diffuser. When the reservoir is empty, repeat if desired.

remedy notes

This recipe may help to inhibit the spread of airborne germs to protect the healthy while relieving sinus congestion for the person who's sick. Above all, this formula banishes the stagnant feelings that set in after being stuck in bed with a cold or sinus infection.

Yarrow and Peppermint Tea

BENEFITS AND USES: *stops a "hot" cold in its early stages*

AVOID: *during pregnancy*

YIELDS: 2 servings

▸ **2 teaspoons dried peppermint leaf**

▸ **2 teaspoons dried yarrow**

▸ **1½ cups hot water**

Place peppermint and yarrow in a tea ball, teapot with strainer, French press, or paper tea filter. Cover with hot water from a recently boiled kettle. Let steep, covered, 15 minutes and then strain and serve.

remedy notes

A "hot" cold is one that includes some or all of the following symptoms: sudden onset of symptoms, feeling warm, running a fever, strong thirst with a desire for cold beverages, and a yellow coating on a bright red tongue. If you catch it in the earliest stage and use a cooling diaphoretic formula like this one, you can sometimes stop the cold in its tracks. Drink as much of this tea as possible during the first 24 hours of your cold while wrapped in warm clothes and blankets to encourage sweating.

✈ Ginger and Turmeric Tea ✈

BENEFITS AND USES: *stops a "cold" cold in its early stages*

AVOID: *during pregnancy or in combination with blood thinners*

YIELDS: 4 servings

- 1 teaspoon ground turmeric
- ⅛ teaspoon ground black pepper
- 3 cups water, divided
- ¼ cup peeled and diced fresh ginger root

1 Add turmeric and black pepper to a medium pot along with 1 tablespoon of the water. Cook over medium heat, stirring constantly, until mixture looks like a creamy paste, about 4 minutes.

2 Add the diced ginger root along with remaining water and bring up to a simmer. Simmer for 15 minutes, strain, and serve.

remedy notes

A "cold" cold is one that includes some or all of the following symptoms: slow onset of symptoms, feeling cold or chilled, a low-grade or no fever at all, runny nose with clear or white mucus, and a thick white tongue coating. If you catch it in the earliest stage and use a warming, sweat-inducing formula like this one, you can sometimes stop the cold in its tracks. Drink as much of this tea as possible during the first 24 hours of your cold while wrapped in warm clothes and blankets to encourage sweating.

❧ Sage and Licorice ❧
Sore Throat Soother

BENEFITS AND USES: *soothes an inflamed sore throat due to an acute strep or upper respiratory infection*

AVOID: *during pregnancy, if breastfeeding, if you have hypertension, or if you're taking corticosteroids*

YIELDS: 2 servings

▸ ½ teaspoon dried licorice root

▸ 1½ cups water

▸ 2 teaspoons dried sage

1 Combine licorice root and water in a small pot over high heat. Bring to a boil and then decrease heat to a simmer. Simmer for 10–15 minutes.

2 Add sage to the pot and turn off the heat. Cover and steep 10 more minutes. Strain and serve. Drink 4–6 ounces as needed throughout the day to relieve cough and sore throat.

 remedy notes

In large amounts, licorice can cause water retention and raise blood pressure. Licorice increases the effects of corticosteroid medications, so if you're taking prednisone, do not use licorice without the guidance of an experienced practitioner. If you'd like, you can replace the licorice with 1 teaspoon marshmallow root and 1 teaspoon mullein leaf.

✈ Elderberry Tea ✦

BENEFITS AND USES: *reduces the severity and duration of a viral infection like the flu or common cold*

AVOID: *if you have an autoimmune disorder and are concerned about using elderberries*

YIELDS: 2 servings

▸ ⅛ **cup dried elderberries**

▸ **2 cups water**

1 Combine elderberries and water in a small, heavy-bottomed pot. Bring to a boil and then decrease to a gentle simmer. Simmer until tea is colorful and fragrant, about 15 minutes.

2 Strain and serve. Serve hot if you're experiencing a runny nose, flu-like symptoms, or chills. Serve over ice if you're drinking it for prevention or pleasure.

remedy notes

Antibiotics don't help with the common cold or the flu, but if your doctor tells you there's nothing she can do for you, that doesn't mean you're stuck! Drink this tea liberally for the best chance at a quick recovery. If desired, sweeten with a splash of orange juice.

Ginger Honey Lemon Tea

YIELDS: 4 servings

- ½ cup peeled and thinly sliced fresh ginger root
- 4 cups water
- Juice of 1 large lemon (about 3 tablespoons)
- ¼ cup raw honey

1 Add ginger and water to a small, heavy-bottomed pot and simmer over medium heat for 30 minutes or until the whole kitchen is fragrant and the water has turned a light golden color.

2 Turn off the heat and add lemon juice and honey. Taste the tea and adjust the flavors to your liking, if needed, by adding more honey or lemon juice. Strain and serve.

remedy notes

The warming and pungent properties of the ginger root relieve congestion, while the sourness of the lemon helps to astringe swollen, boggy tissue. Honey balances the formula with humectant properties that rehydrate the throat and stop coughing. This decoction can also increase your energy on cold mornings when you're feeling sluggish and don't want to get out of bed.

Immune-Boosting Broth with Shiitake and Astragalus

BENEFITS AND USES: *helps you stay healthy and energetic during cold and flu season*

AVOID: *if you're already sick; check with your practitioner if taking immunosuppressant medication or blood thinners*

YIELDS: 12 servings

- 2 tablespoons olive oil
- 2 large onions, peeled and diced
- 4 carrots, diced
- 4 stalks celery, ends removed and diced
- 8 garlic cloves, smashed and skins removed
- 10 sprigs fresh thyme
- 2 sprigs fresh rosemary
- 2 bay leaves
- 4 quarts water
- 8 ounces fresh shiitake mushrooms, sliced (or 4 ounces dried, soaked in water to rehydrate)
- 12 slices dried astragalus root
- 4 tablespoons nutritional yeast
- ½ cup miso paste, divided (2 teaspoons per serving)

---

1 Coat the bottom of a large stockpot with oil and warm over medium heat. Once oil is warm, add onions, carrots, and celery.

2 Cook over medium heat 6–7 minutes, stirring occasionally to ensure that veggies are coated with oil and cooking evenly. When veggies are fragrant and soft, add garlic and cook another 1–2 minutes.

3 Using cheesecloth and clean kitchen twine, tie thyme and rosemary sprigs into a bundle.

4 Add water, cheesecloth herb bundle, mushrooms (along with the soaking water, if you used dried shiitakes), and astragalus slices to the pot. Cover. Turn the heat to high and bring to a boil. Once boiling, turn down the heat to medium and partially uncover the pot. Simmer, partially covered, 30 minutes and then add nutritional yeast.

5 Remove the astragalus and herb bundle from the broth. Strain the veggies out, if desired. If not using right away, store broth in the fridge 4–5 days, or in the freezer 3–4 months.

6 To serve, spoon 2 teaspoons miso paste into each serving vessel—mugs, teacups, and bowls all work well. Ladle 1 cup hot broth over miso paste, using the back of a spoon to help paste dissolve completely into broth. Drink and enjoy.

remedy notes

Astragalus strengthens the immune system to improve your resistance to infection. It's often sold in slices that resemble tongue depressors, which makes it easy to remove from any finished recipe. Throughout cold and flu season, add a few strips of astragalus to any soup or stock you make. The flavor is mellow; it won't affect the finished dish.

⤞ Classic Fire Cider ⤝

BENEFITS AND USES: *keeps your immune system in tip-top shape during cold-weather months*

AVOID: *if you have gastroesophageal reflux disease (GERD) that's triggered by spicy food and/or vinegar. Ask your doctor before using if you're taking blood thinners.*

YIELDS: about 3 cups

- ¾ cup freshly grated horseradish root
- 1 medium onion, peeled and roughly chopped
- ½ cup garlic cloves, smashed, peeled, and chopped
- ½ cup peeled and chopped fresh ginger root
- 2 fresh chili peppers, halved and seeded
- 1 tablespoon ground turmeric
- 2½ cups apple cider vinegar
- 1 cup raw honey

1 Add the horseradish, onion, garlic, ginger, and chili peppers to a clean quart-sized Mason jar. Add the turmeric, followed by the apple cider vinegar. Cover with a plastic lid and label the jar. (Metal canning lids tend to corrode when exposed to vinegar.)

2 Set aside at least 3 weeks to steep, but you can leave it in a cupboard for up to 2 months if your schedule requires it. Shake the jar a few times a week, if possible!

3 After at least 3 weeks of steeping, strain the infused vinegar through a fine-mesh sieve into a second quart-sized Mason jar. Reserve the solids to make Rosemary's Fire Cider Chutney (see recipe in this chapter). Add honey to the infused vinegar and stir to combine. The finished product will keep in the fridge at least 6 months and up to a year.

4 To use, take ½ tablespoon per day during the winter months as a general tonic. Before a meal is best. If you feel yourself getting sick, increase the dose to ½ tablespoon a few times per day.

✦ Rosemary's Fire Cider Chutney ✦

BENEFITS AND USES: *supports your immune system and digestion*

AVOID: *if you have gastroesophageal reflux disease (GERD) that's triggered by spicy food and/or vinegar. Ask your doctor before use if you're taking blood thinners.*

YIELDS: about 2½ cups

- 4 medjool dates
- ½ cup water
- Reserved solid ingredients from Classic Fire Cider (see recipe in this chapter), about 2 cups
- 2 teaspoons Turmeric Paste (see Chapter 8)
- 1 tablespoon raw honey

1 Soak the dates overnight in ½ cup water. Remove the pits and add dates to the bowl of your food processor along with 2 tablespoons of the soaking water. Process until the dates form a smooth paste, about 4 minutes.

2 Add the reserved Classic Fire Cider solid ingredients and the Turmeric Paste to the date mixture. Pulse for 2 seconds at a time for a total of 1–2 minutes until the mixture forms an evenly chunky paste.

3 Add raw honey and stir to combine.

4 Store in the refrigerator in a covered container for up to 2 weeks.

remedy notes

I'm sharing this recipe in honor of Rosemary Gladstar, the herbalist who first created something called "fire cider" and a version of this chutney. Recipes like these have been passed down for generations, and Rosemary has worked hard to make sure that private companies don't trademark classic recipes for private gain. This chutney is delicious served on whole grains, over warm beans, alongside meat, or paired with creamy avocado on toast.

⇻ Elderberry Spice Syrup ⇺

YIELDS: about 4 cups

- 1 organic lemon
- 1 cup dried elderberries
- 5 cups water
- ¼ cup peeled and sliced fresh ginger root
- ½ tablespoon whole cloves
- 1 cinnamon stick
- About 2 cups raw honey

1 Peel lemon and cut peel into strips. Juice lemon into a small bowl and set aside.

2 Add lemon peel, elderberries, water, ginger, cloves, and cinnamon stick to a medium, heavy-bottomed pot. Bring to a boil and then turn down the heat to a simmer. Allow the mixture to simmer gently 25 minutes or until the liquid is dark and the volume has reduced by about ⅓. Turn off heat and allow to cool slightly.

3 Strain liquid (it's now a decoction) through a fine-mesh sieve and some cheesecloth, squeezing berries to extract as much liquid as possible. Discard the spent berries.

4 Add fresh lemon juice to the elderberry decoction. Measure the volume of the liquid and add an equal amount of raw honey to turn the decoction into elderberry syrup.

5 To use, take ½ tablespoon three times per day at the first signs of a viral infection. Store the finished syrup in the refrigerator up to 3 months.

Rosemary and Thyme Oxymel

BENEFITS AND USES: *relieves a productive cough accompanied by chest congestion and throat irritation*

AVOID: *if you have gastroesophageal reflux disease (GERD) that's triggered by spicy food and/or vinegar*

YIELDS: about ¾ cup
- **2 tablespoons dried rosemary**
- **2 tablespoons dried thyme**
- **2 tablespoons water**
- **½ cup plus 2 tablespoons apple cider vinegar**
- **½ cup raw honey**

1 Add rosemary, thyme, and water to a small pot. Warm over medium-low heat about 5 minutes, stirring constantly, until herbs absorb the water.

2 As soon as herbs absorb the water, add apple cider vinegar and bring the mixture to a low simmer. Partially cover the pot with a lid and continue to simmer gently for 10 minutes. Turn off heat and cover with the lid. Let stand on the burner, covered, 10 minutes.

3 Strain through a fine-mesh sieve into a clean bowl or Mason jar and discard spent herbs. Add honey and stir until honey softens and dissolves. If honey doesn't incorporate easily into vinegar, wipe out the pot with a clean towel to remove any remaining herbs. Then warm the honey and vinegar mixture over low heat until incorporated. Bottle finished oxymel in a pint-sized Mason jar fitted with a plastic lid and a clear label. Store at room temperature up to 6 months.

4 To use, take ½ tablespoon as needed when you have an upper respiratory infection and a productive cough.

⊷ Smashed Garlic Tea ⊶

BENEFITS AND USES: *prevents and relieves a secondary bronchial infection after a cold or the flu*

AVOID: *if you're taking blood thinners or suffer from heartburn*

YIELDS: 1 cup

➤ **1 large garlic clove, smashed and peeled**

➤ **1 cup hot water**

Place bruised garlic clove in your favorite teacup or mug. Pour hot water over garlic and cover cup with a saucer. Let steep 10–15 minutes and stir before drinking.

Your body eliminates the sulfur compounds in garlic and onions through the lungs. On their way out, these compounds have significant power to limit the growth of bacteria in the bronchi. If you don't like the idea of drinking garlic tea, you can incorporate a clove or two of raw garlic into your food (try the Garlic Gremolata in Chapter 8!) for the same benefits.

✈ Mullein Tea ✈

BENEFITS AND USES: *comforts a sore throat, quiets a dry cough, and helps to revive a hoarse, raspy voice*

AVOID: *if you're taking blood thinners, unless your doctor gives you personalized advice on safe use*

YIELDS: 1 cup

▸ **1 scant tablespoon dried mullein leaf**

▸ **1 cup hot water**

1 Add mullein leaf to a paper tea filter, large tea ball, or other container designed to brew loose-leaf tea. Drop tea bag or ball into your favorite teacup.

2 Pour hot water over herb and let steep at least 10 minutes. Drink liberally until you're feeling better.

Mullein is a demulcent and an expectorant, so it's capable of both hydrating irritated tissue and helping you to cough up anything that's stuck in your lungs. It's a great addition to any tea blend for colds, coughs, and upper respiratory infections. Add ½ tablespoon dried peppermint leaf to this tea if you need something to change the flavor, or 1 tablespoon dried catnip if you're taking this at bedtime and need some help to relax.

Lobelia Tincture for Asthma and Dry Coughs

BENEFITS AND USES: *releases bronchospasm and relaxes all of the involuntary muscles of the chest*

AVOID: *taking more than the recommended amount; if you're pregnant; combining with blood pressure medication, bronchodilators, sedatives, psychotropic medication, anti-seizure medication, or blood thinners*

YIELDS: 50+ applications

▸ 1 (1-ounce) bottle *Lobelia inflata* tincture (see Chapter 2 for detailed information on where to purchase herbs)

▸ ⅛ cup water

1 *Determine your dose:* Place 5 drops of the tincture in water and drink. Wait 5 minutes and notice how you feel. If your chest seems to open up, your breathing gets easier, and you feel slightly relaxed, great! In that case, 5 drops is a good dose for you. If you feel nothing, take 10 more drops in a little bit of water. Wait another 5 minutes. If you get the desired results, 15 drops is a good dose for you. If you feel nothing, try another 10 drops. Once you take a dose that creates a relaxing effect, write a note on the bottle so you'll remember how much to take. Do not exceed ½ teaspoon or 50 drops of tincture in one sitting. If you feel nauseated, do not use the tincture again for 24 hours.

Lobelia Tincture for Asthma and Dry Coughs—continued

2 *To use:* When experiencing a dry, barking, asthmatic cough, take the dose of Lobelia tincture that you figured out in the first step. If you have asthma symptoms that are triggered by cold air or exercise, take a dose before stepping out into cold air or before a workout to prevent the problem before it starts. Do not exceed 1 teaspoon of the tincture in a 24-hour period unless advised to do so by an experienced practitioner.

remedy notes

Lobelia is also a wonderful remedy for stress, insomnia, and anxiety. It is considered a "parasympathomimetic" remedy because it has the power to activate the parasympathetic branch of your nervous system. The parasympathetic nervous system is the opposite of the stress response that encourages you to "fight or flee." Lobelia helps you to rest, digest your food, and feel safe. Lobelia can help relieve anxiety and tension without causing sedation, and it can even work as an aphrodisiac for people who feel too stressed out to get in the mood for lovemaking. I'll confess: it's my favorite herb.

Poke Root Lymphatic Oil
with Rosemary and Lemon Balm

BENEFITS AND USES: *relieves lymphatic congestion, swelling, and soreness when you're sick*

AVOID: *if pregnant or breastfeeding; do not use internally, and keep away from children and pets*

YIELDS: about 1 cup

- 1 cup unrefined sesame oil
- ½ cup washed, dried, and chopped fresh poke root
- 20 drops rosemary essential oil
- ½ teaspoon 10 percent dilution lemon balm essential oil (or 20 drops of the undiluted essential oil)

1 Set up a double boiler by adding 3"–4" of warm water to a medium pot and situating a heat-safe glass bowl over the pot so that it isn't touching the water. Place sesame oil and poke root in the glass bowl and turn the burner on low. Warm over low heat for 2 hours, checking every 30 minutes to replenish the water, if needed, and to ensure that the oil doesn't get too hot. (It's getting too hot if bubbles start to form. If that happens, turn off heat and let the mixture cool 30 minutes before reapplying heat.) After 2 hours of infusing, let stand until cool enough to handle.

2 Strain through a fine-mesh sieve lined with cheesecloth into a small bowl or liquid measuring cup. Make sure to give the cheesecloth a good squeeze with your hands to extract as much of the medicated oil as possible. Dispose of spent poke root so that pets and children won't find it; it could make them sick if they ingest it.

Poke Root Lymphatic Oil with Rosemary and Lemon Balm—continued

3 Add the essential oils to the infused sesame oil and stir once or twice to combine. Pour the finished oil into a pint-sized Mason jar or 2 (4-ounce) bottles of your choice. Clearly label each bottle "Do not drink." Store at room temperature and use within 1 year.

4 To use oil, apply 1 teaspoon twice per day to the areas with a high concentration of lymph nodes, including the neck, armpits, and inner thigh/groin (avoiding the genital region). Be gentle and use very light pressure since these are delicate areas of your body. Spend extra time on any areas that feel sore or congested.

remedy notes

Your lymphatic system gets congested when you're sick because it's flooded with immune cells and waste products that need to move to and from the affected tissues. This oil can help relieve some of the lymphatic "traffic jam" and facilitate your overall recovery. For even better results, watch a video or two to learn the basic techniques of lymphatic massage and use them whenever you apply this oil.

Echinacea Tincture for Immune Support

BENEFITS AND USES: *helps your body fight bacterial infections*

AVOID: *if you're taking antibiotics or blood thinners*

YIELDS: about 1 cup

- ¾ **cup dried root of** *Echinacea angustifolia* **or** *Echinacea purpurea*
- **3 cups 100-proof vodka**
- **Water**

1 Add echinacea root and vodka to a pint- or quart-sized Mason jar and cover with a lid. Shake well. Label the jar and let stand on the counter for 4 weeks, shaking once per day.

2 After 4 weeks, the tincture will be ready. Strain through a fine-mesh sieve into a clean pint-sized Mason jar. Cover and label the jar with the date and the ingredients. The tincture will keep for 5 years if stored at cool room temperature.

3 *To prevent illness or to prevent a sinus or bronchial infection from developing when you're already sick:* Take ¼ teaspoon tincture in water (at least ⅛ cup, but feel free to dilute with more water if you prefer) twice per day. Limit preventive use to no longer than 2 weeks.

4 *If you have a sinus infection, urinary tract infection, or bronchial infection in the very early stage:* Take ½ teaspoon tincture in water (at least ⅛ cup, but feel free to dilute with more water if you prefer). Then take another ¼ teaspoon tincture in water every hour while you're awake. Drink lots of fluids and let yourself rest to maximize the efficacy of the herb.

 remedy notes

Echinacea is best for internal use when you're feeling overheated or feverish; have a red tongue with a yellowish coating; have yellow or green mucus when you blow your nose or cough up phlegm; and/or the pulse on the inside of your wrist (radial pulse) is fast and force-ful. Echinacea is also a great herb for skin infections. Apply the tincture two to three times per day directly to cuts, scrapes, infected bug bites, or sores that are producing yellowish pus.

Chapter 6

DIGESTIVE HEALTH

Cultivating great digestion is a little bit like cooking a delicious meal. While it's possible to slap something together quickly to get the job done, the process benefits from an unhurried pace that indulges all five senses. A purely mechanical approach will always fall short. For great cooking and great digestion alike, pleasure is central.

This chapter includes remedies to enhance and support optimal digestion at every stage of the process. You'll learn to make your own digestive bitters so you can stimulate bile flow and enjoy maximal absorption of the nutrients in your food. You'll learn how simple teas like Tangerine Zest Tea and Cardamom After-Dinner Tea can provide relief from indigestion and how to relieve acid reflux with a Soothing Marshmallow Root Infusion. And you'll learn how to make an inexpensive, gentle remedy for constipation using nothing but whole flaxseed and water. It's gentle enough for children and powerful enough to work in cases of opioid-induced constipation.

Health-conscious people in the modern world tend to be very focused on what to eat. As important as the content of your diet is, how you eat (and how you feel about it) matters at least as much. I hope the remedies in this chapter will support you in learning how to take the time to appreciate and enjoy each meal. Eating slowly, chewing thoroughly, and enjoying nourishing food in a relaxed environment provide the foundation of digestive health. If you need more digestive support, the remedies in this chapter will make a big difference.

❧ Cooling Dandelion Bitters ❧

BENEFITS AND USES: *activates bile flow and improves bile quality*

AVOID: *if your primary digestive symptoms include bloating, lack of appetite, weight loss, aversion to cold food and drinks, and are accompanied by general coldness*

YIELDS: about 2 cups

▸ ⅓ **cup dried dandelion root**

▸ ⅓ **cup fennel seeds**

▸ ⅓ **cup dried peppermint leaf**

▸ **3 cups 100-proof vodka**

1. Combine herbs in a quart-sized Mason jar. Stir to mix.

2. Pour vodka over other ingredients and stir with a knife or chopstick. Label the jar with the date and the ingredients. Secure the lid and set aside for 24 hours.

3. Check on your bitters. The ingredients may have swollen as they absorbed the alcohol while steeping. If there's room at the top of the jar, top it off with another ½ cup vodka after 24–48 hours.

4. Let ingredients steep in the alcohol 2–3 weeks. Shake the jar a few times a week and add a little more vodka, as needed, to keep the ingredients fully submerged.

5. After 3 weeks, strain the bitters through a fine-mesh sieve lined with cheesecloth or unbleached paper towels. Use clean hands to squeeze as much alcohol from the spent ingredients as you can. Bottle in a Mason jar and label with the date and the ingredients. Store away from extreme temperatures and out of reach of children. Bitters will maintain full potency for about 3 years but will still be safe to consume for up to 5 years.

6. *To optimize digestion:* Take ¼ teaspoon in a small amount of water (about ⅛ cup) about 30 minutes before meals.

7. *To relieve indigestion:* Take ½ teaspoon every 30 minutes until symptoms subside.

Fresh Dandelion Leaves for Digestion

BENEFITS AND USES: *encourages good digestion and stimulates appetite*

AVOID: *N/A*

YIELDS: 1 serving

> **3–5 raw dandelion leaves**

Pick dandelion leaves in an area that hasn't been treated with pesticides or herbicides. Fifteen minutes before a meal, wash leaves and eat them. Make sure to chew them thoroughly to activate your digestion and stimulate bile flow. If you find some dandelions on a walk and want to use them later in the day, set them on a napkin or in a small bowl and store at room temperature up to 12 hours. Avoid washing them until just before you're ready to consume them.

When they're young and tender, raw dandelion leaves also make a nutritious addition to any green salad. Wash them and pat them dry after harvesting, and then add to your salad bowl. Top with Golden Ginger Dressing (see Chapter 9) and enjoy!

Warming Chamomile Berry Bitters

BENEFITS AND USES: *soothes indigestion, relieves gas, and optimizes digestion*

AVOID: *if your primary digestive symptoms are made worse by spicy food*

YIELDS: about 2 cups

- ⅓ cup dried chamomile flowers
- ¼ cup dried hawthorn berries
- ½ cup water
- 1 tablespoon grated organic orange zest
- 1 tablespoon grated fresh ginger root
- 1 cinnamon stick
- 3 cups 80-proof white rum

1 Add chamomile flowers, hawthorn berries, and water to a small pot and bring to a simmer over moderate heat, stirring constantly. Cook for 6–7 minutes, until berries have plumped up slightly and all of the water has been absorbed.

2 Combine warm, slightly damp berry mixture with the orange zest, ginger root, and cinnamon stick in a quart-sized Mason jar.

3 Pour rum over the mixture and stir. Cover and set aside 24 hours.

4 Check on your bitters after 24 hours. The herbs may have swollen as they absorbed the alcohol while steeping. If there's room at the top of the jar, top it off with another ½ cup rum after 24–48 hours.

5 Let ingredients steep 2–3 weeks. Shake the jar a few times a week, adding more rum, as needed, to keep the ingredients fully submerged.

Warming Chamomile Berry Bitters—continued

6 After 3 weeks, strain the bitters through a fine-mesh sieve lined with cheesecloth or unbleached paper towels. Use clean hands to squeeze as much alcohol from the spent ingredients as you can. Bottle in a Mason jar and label with the date and the ingredients. Store away from extreme temperatures and out of reach of children. Bitters will maintain full potency for about 3 years but will still be safe to consume for up to five years.

7 *To optimize digestion:* Take 1 teaspoon in a small amount of water (about ⅛ cup) 30 minutes before meals.

8 *To relieve indigestion:* Take ½ teaspoon every 30 minutes until symptoms subside.

remedy notes

This recipe is best for people with "cold" constitutions who tend toward timidity, feeling cold, low appetite, and slow digestion. This recipe is for you if you fit some of those descriptors and your digestive woes tend toward lack of appetite, fear of how your body will respond if you eat the wrong foods, bloating after eating, or feeling like food sits in your stomach for a long time after a meal.

Chocolate Spice Bitters

BENEFITS AND USES: *increases appetite and encourages good digestion*

AVOID: *if you are very sensitive to caffeine or if chocolate triggers headaches*

YIELDS: about 2 cups

- ⅓ **cup cacao nibs**
- ⅓ **cup cardamom pods**
- **1 tablespoon grated organic orange zest**
- **3 cups 80-proof white rum**

1 Combine cacao nibs, cardamom pods, and orange zest in a quart-sized Mason jar.

2 Pour rum over the top and stir with a knife or chopstick. Cover and set aside for 24 hours.

3 Let ingredients steep in alcohol at least 3 weeks. Shake the jar a few times a week and add a little more rum, as needed, to keep ingredients fully submerged.

4 After 3 weeks, strain bitters through a fine-mesh sieve lined with cheesecloth or unbleached paper towels. Use clean hands to squeeze as much alcohol from the spent ingredients as you can. Bottle in a Mason jar and label with the date and the ingredients. Store away from extreme temperatures and out of reach of children. These bitters will maintain full potency for about 1 year but will still be safe to consume for up to 3 years.

5 *To optimize digestion:* Take 1 teaspoon in a small amount of water (about ⅛ cup) about 30 minutes before meals.

6 *To relieve indigestion:* Take ½ teaspoon every 30 minutes until symptoms subside.

⇥ Hawthorn Berry Cooler ↤

BENEFITS AND USES: *encourages good digestion and supplies your body with vitamin C and antioxidants*

AVOID: *N/A*

YIELDS: about 3 cups

- ½ cup dried hawthorn berries
- ¼ cup dried rose hips
- 4 cups water
- 1 tablespoon raw honey
- 1 cup ice cubes

1 Add hawthorn berries, rose hips, and water to a medium, heavy-bottomed pot and bring to a boil. Reduce heat to a simmer and partially cover. Let simmer 20 minutes.

2 Strain the tea through a fine-mesh sieve into a heat-safe pitcher. Make sure to squeeze the spent berries and rose hips to extract as much water as possible before discarding. Stir in honey right away, while the tea is still warm.

3 Add ice. Serve chilled as an iced tea to support digestion during hot weather.

remedy notes

Hawthorn berries have abundant benefits for cardiovascular health as well as digestion, and rose hips are full of antioxidants. This preparation is ideal for people with risk factors for heart disease who want to optimize their digestion and support cardiovascular health at the same time.

⊱ Emergency Baking Soda Antacid ⊰

BENEFITS AND USES: *calms heartburn or acid reflux when there are no other remedies available*

AVOID: *if you have high blood pressure or are on a low-sodium diet; using more than the recommended dose*

YIELDS: 1 serving

➤ ½ **teaspoon baking soda**

➤ ¾ **cup water**

Stir baking soda into a 6-ounce glass of water and drink.

Baking soda (sodium bicarbonate) has an alkaline pH and should help to relieve symptoms of acid reflux within 5–10 minutes of drinking this remedy. It works well in a pinch; just don't use this on a regular basis. Too much sodium in any form can cause water retention and raise blood pressure; baking soda is no exception.

Soothing Marshmallow Root Infusion

BENEFITS AND USES: *relieves the discomfort of acid reflux and heals the esophagus after chronic exposure to stomach acid*

AVOID: *taking other medications less than 1 hour before (or 4 hours after) drinking this infusion*

YIELDS: 4 servings

> ⅓ cup marshmallow root
> 4 cups room temperature water

1 Add marshmallow root to a quart-sized Mason jar. Fill the jar with water and cover with a lid. Shake or stir until all of the marshmallow root is saturated with water. Let it infuse at room temperature for 4–8 hours or overnight.

2 Using cheesecloth or a nut milk bag, strain the pale golden infusion to separate the liquid from the solid marshmallow root pieces. Make sure to thoroughly squeeze the remaining root to get out as much of the gel-like liquid (called mucilage) that's full of concentrated soothing power as you can. Discard the used roots.

3 To use, stir infusion well. Drink 1 cup (or more) as needed to relieve heartburn. If you have chronic acid reflux, drink 2–4 cups throughout the day to support tissue healing in your esophagus.

4 Store leftover infusion in a covered container in the refrigerator and consume within 48 hours. Stir well before pouring yourself a serving since the beneficial compounds tend to settle at the bottom of the jar or pitcher after a few hours.

⊹ Tangerine Zest Tea ⊹

BENEFITS AND USES: *drink before or with meals to prevent indigestion, curb overeating, and/or relieve the feeling of food "just sitting there" after a meal*

AVOID: *if you can't access organic citrus or if you're allergic*

YIELDS: 1 cup
- ½ teaspoon grated organic tangerine zest
- ¾ cup hot water

1 Place zest at the bottom of a teacup. Pour hot water over the zest. Cover the cup with a saucer to keep the steam from escaping. (This prevents the essential oils from evaporating.)

2 Let tea steep 10–15 minutes. Sip slowly, either before your meal or as you eat.

remedy notes

Chinese medicine teaches that various kinds of citrus peel affect the body's vital energy in different ways, but the thing they share in common is that they relieve stagnation. As you drink this tea, notice how you feel. Can you sense any subtle movement or release in your body or mind? You can substitute orange, clementine, lemon, or lime zest. Just make sure it's organic since agricultural chemicals are hard to remove from the rind even if you wash your fruit. Dried citrus peel will work, but it won't be quite as potent.

Fennel Seed "Quick Fix"

BENEFITS AND USES: *sweetens your breath and prevents gas and bloating*

AVOID: *N/A*

YIELDS: 1 serving

> 2 teaspoons fennel seeds

Chew seeds thoroughly after a meal that could cause bad breath, gas, or indigestion. Repeat as needed.

remedy notes

Fennel relaxes involuntary muscle spasms in the digestive tract and relieves gas, which is why it's so effective for indigestion and irritable bowel syndrome (IBS). Since these actions come from the essential oils, which degrade quickly, choose fennel seeds that are fragrant and green. Store fennel seeds in an airtight container away from light and extreme temperatures to preserve their efficacy.

✈ Instant Ginger Lemon Tea ✦

BENEFITS AND USES: *stimulates digestion or calms an upset stomach*

AVOID: *if you have gastroesophageal reflux disease (GERD) that's triggered by sour or spicy foods or if you're taking blood thinners*

YIELDS: 1 cup

➤ ¼ teaspoon grated fresh ginger root

➤ 1 cup hot water

➤ 1 tablespoon freshly squeezed lemon juice

1 Place ginger at the bottom of a teacup. Cover with hot water.

2 Cover the cup with a saucer and let the ginger steep 5 minutes.

3 Just before serving, add freshly squeezed lemon juice.

remedy notes

Fresh ginger has a warm, pungent flavor as well as anti-inflammatory properties. At the dose suggested in this recipe, it's helpful for cases of mild constipation, slow digestion, or the discomfort that arises from overindulging. It's also a wonderful remedy for nausea. Grating the ginger makes it possible for this tea to be ready quickly. If desired, you can sweeten to taste with honey, maple syrup, or a splash of orange juice.

Simplest Apple Cider Vinegar Tonic

BENEFITS AND USES: *optimizes blood sugar response and supports better insulin sensitivity*

AVOID: *if you have gastroesophageal reflux disease (GERD) or acid reflux that's triggered by vinegar*

YIELDS: 1 serving

> 1 tablespoon apple cider vinegar
> 1 cup water

1 Stir apple cider vinegar into water.

2 Drink the full glass of vinegar/water mixture within 15 minutes.

remedy notes

This is one of those remedies that seems too good to be true, but there are a number of scientific studies that support apple cider vinegar's ability to promote insulin sensitivity and improved blood sugar levels for people with metabolic syndrome. Effective home remedies don't get any simpler or more affordable than this! Apple cider vinegar has been shown to reduce fasting blood sugar, improve insulin response, and support weight loss. In the studies that showed these benefits, participants consumed 1–2 tablespoons apple cider vinegar multiple times per day for many weeks. As with any good habit, being consistent is the key to good results.

Herbal Mouthwash

BENEFITS AND USES: *supports a healthy oral environment; prevents and helps to reverse gum disease*

AVOID: *if you have an autoimmune condition and/or respond poorly to echinacea*

YIELDS: about 60 applications

- ⅛ cup dried sage
- ⅛ cup dried yarrow
- ⅛ cup dried calendula flowers
- ⅛ cup dried peppermint leaf
- ¼ cup dried echinacea root
- ¼ cup fresh plantain leaves, wilted and finely chopped (see Chapter 2)
- 3 cups (80–90-proof) vodka
- ⅛ cup water, per use

---

1 Combine herbs in a quart-sized Mason jar.

2 Pour vodka over herbs. Close the jar with a tight-fitting lid and shake well.

3 Let herbs steep at room temperature for 4 weeks. Shake the jar at least three times per week (daily, if you can!) while steeping to facilitate the process.

4 When the concentrate is done steeping, drape a double layer of cheesecloth over a funnel. Place the cheesecloth-lined funnel over another clean quart-sized Mason jar. Strain the herb and vodka mixture through the cheesecloth. Use your hands to squeeze as much liquid from the spent herbs as you can before discarding the herb material and the cheesecloth.

5 Label the finished concentrate and store at room temperature out of reach of children. The concentrate will have full potency for 3 years but will still be safe to use for up to 5 years.

6 To use, mix ½ tablespoon concentrate with about ⅛ cup water. Swish around your mouth for at least 1 minute. For best results, use twice per day after brushing and flossing.

⇥ Cardamom After-Dinner Tea ⇤

BENEFITS AND USES: *relieves mild gas and indigestion*

AVOID: *N/A*

YIELDS: 1 serving

- ▸ **6 green cardamom pods**
- ▸ **1 black tea bag of choice (decaf or regular)**
- ▸ **¾ cup hot water**

1 Add cardamom pods and tea bag to a teacup and cover with hot water.

2 Cover the cup with a saucer and steep at least 5 minutes.

Cardamom's aromatic compounds are not only delicious: they're also one of the best ways to settle your stomach after a meal. This tea can also satisfy the urge for something sweet at the end of a meal if you feel the need for a treat but don't have room for dessert. In fact, you can sweeten this tea with a teaspoon of maple syrup or honey for even more of a treat. A splash of almond milk pairs beautifully with cardamom too.

⤙ Peppermint and Fennel IBS Relief ⤚

BENEFITS AND USES: *relieves gas, bloating, and abdominal discomfort associated with irritable bowel syndrome (IBS)*

AVOID: *N/A*

YIELDS: 4 servings

➤ ⅛ cup fennel seeds

➤ ¼ cup dried peppermint leaf

➤ 4 cups hot water

1 Crush fennel seeds with a mortar and pestle, or by enclosing them in a zip-top bag and rolling back and forth over the bag with a rolling pin a few times. Add crushed fennel seeds and peppermint to a quart-sized Mason jar. Cover the herbs with hot water.

2 Cover the top of the jar with a saucer to prevent the aromatic compounds from escaping as the tea steeps. Let steep 15 minutes.

3 Strain and drink, as needed. Store any leftovers in a covered container in the refrigerator and drink within 48 hours. Leftovers are great as an iced tea, but you can warm them up and drink them hot too.

 remedy notes

This formula addresses the painful cramping and intestinal gas that can be associated with some forms of irritable bowel syndrome (IBS). If you have IBS, one of the best things you can do is figure out your triggers and avoid them as often as possible. A good probiotic supplement can also help.

Chamomile and Calendula Gut Healer

BENEFITS AND USES: *relieves gas, bloating, and indigestion while healing gut lining damage*

AVOID: *using licorice if you have high blood pressure or are taking prednisone; substitute ⅛ cup crushed fennel seeds instead*

YIELDS: 4 servings

- ⅛ cup dried chamomile flowers
- ¼ cup dried calendula flowers
- ¼ cup dried peppermint leaf
- 1 heaping teaspoon dried licorice root
- 4 cups hot water

1 Add herbs to a quart-sized Mason jar. Cover with hot water.

2 Cover the top of the jar with a saucer to prevent the aromatic compounds from escaping as the tea steeps. Let steep 20 minutes.

3 Strain through cheesecloth or a fine-mesh sieve and drink. Keep leftovers in the fridge up to 48 hours.

remedy notes

Healing your gut does take some dedication, but it doesn't have to be complicated. A good starting protocol would be to drink two servings of this formula per day for 3 weeks. During that 3-week period, avoid foods that trigger your symptoms and take a high-potency probiotic supplement.

Happy Belly Massage Oil

BENEFITS AND USES: *relieves abdominal tension and discomfort and prevents/relieves mild constipation*

AVOID: *during pregnancy*

YIELDS: 12 applications

- **20 drops Roman chamomile essential oil**
- **7 drops geranium essential oil**
- **5 drops clary sage essential oil**
- **5 drops lavender essential oil**
- **¼ cup plus 2 tablespoons unrefined sesame oil**

1 Add essential oils to a clean jar or bottle that's large enough to hold at least ¼ cup of liquid. Cover with sesame oil and shake well to blend.

2 To use, massage ½ tablespoon of oil onto your abdomen. Start with large, clockwise circles covering the whole belly. After a few minutes of clockwise circles, gently massage the colon to encourage it to empty. Start with the descending colon (on the left side of your body), massaging with slightly deeper pressure from below your left rib cage to the top of your pelvic bowl. Continue with the transverse colon (just below your rib cage), stroking from the right side to the left. Finally, massage the ascending colon with deeper pressure, starting on the inside of the right hip bone and traveling up toward the right rib cage. Finish the massage with a few additional minutes of clockwise circles.

remedy notes

Ayurvedic tradition teaches that the solar plexus is the location of an energy center that has to do with your sense of self, the strength of your will, and your personal power. Abdominal massage is a wonderful way to support this energy center while releasing patterns of tension that interfere with breathing, digestion, and self-confidence.

Miso Broth for Recovery after Diarrhea

BENEFITS AND USES: *eases your body back into eating after a bout of diarrhea*

AVOID: *if drinking this broth causes your symptoms to return*

YIELDS: 1 serving

- ½ **tablespoon unpasteurized miso paste**
- **1 cup hot water**

Stir unpasteurized miso paste into hot water. When drinking, sip very slowly since a large volume of hot liquid can trigger a reflex that will cause you to have a bowel movement.

remedy notes

Once you can tolerate this broth, continue to add bland, low-residue foods back to your diet until you're able to eat normally again. Try the classic BRAT diet: bananas, rice, applesauce, and toast, in addition to this miso broth, and an electrolyte replacement drink (try the Citrus and Sea Salt Electrolyte Replenisher in Chapter 8). If severe diarrhea lasts for more than 48 hours or if you have severe abdominal pain, bleeding, or a very high fever, seek medical treatment.

Cool Raspberry Leaf and Yarrow Tea

BENEFITS AND USES: *firms up loose stools*

AVOID: *if you're taking diuretics or blood thinners*

YIELDS: 1 serving

- **2 teaspoons dried raspberry leaf**
- **1 teaspoon dried yarrow**
- **¾ cup hot water**
- **3 grains sea salt**
- **½ cup ice cubes**

1 Place raspberry and yarrow into a tea strainer, tea ball, paper tea filter, or other vessel for brewing and straining loose-leaf tea. Cover with
  hot water and let steep 15 minutes.

2 Strain the liquid from the spent leaves into a heat-safe cup or mug.
  Add salt and ice cubes and stir until the ice is dissolved. The liquid
  should be room temperature or cooler.

3 Sip the tea very slowly, as needed, to help firm up loose stools.

remedy notes

Raspberry leaf helps to tone and strengthen tissues that have
become boggy, lax, or loose. It's gentle in its astringent action
and a cooling, nourishing tonic at the same time. Yarrow echoes
the uplifting, tonifying, and astringent properties of raspberry but
has a more "warming" nature that brings balance to this formula.
For use during pregnancy, omit the yarrow since it may trigger
uterine contractions.

⊱ Flaxseed Stool Softener ⊰

BENEFITS AND USES: *relieves mild to moderate constipation*

AVOID: *relying on this remedy for more than 2 weeks without consulting a medical professional*

YIELDS: 1 serving

➤ **1 tablespoon whole flaxseed**

➤ **1 cup room temperature water**

1 Add flaxseed to a water glass and cover with water.

2 Stir gently so that all of the seeds are submerged in water. Cover and let sit on the counter or in the fridge at least 4 hours and up to 12 hours. After steeping, the water becomes a gel that can lubricate and soothe your large intestine so that you can have a comfortable bowel movement.

3 To serve, stir once or twice and then strain through a fine-mesh sieve, nut milk bag, or cheesecloth into a glass. Reserve the soaked seeds for another recipe if desired. Drink immediately, and use any reserved flaxseed within 24 hours.

4 The resulting flax water is the medicinal substance. Drink it. After drinking one glass, start another batch. Continue making and drinking the flax water twice per day until you're having regular, comfortable bowel movements.

remedy notes

This is the safest and most effective stool softener I know. It's gentle enough for people with sensitive digestive systems yet powerful enough to combat opioid-induced constipation. If your constipation is mild, you may have a bowel movement within 8–12 hours of your first dose. If not, continue drinking the remedy twice per day until you're consistently having satisfying bowel movements on a daily basis.

Witch Hazel and Yarrow Pads

BENEFITS AND USES: *reduces pain, swelling, and bleeding associated with hemorrhoids*

AVOID: *relying on this remedy for more than 2 weeks without consulting a medical professional*

YIELDS: about 30 pads

- ¼ cup dried yarrow
- ¼ cup dried plantain leaf
- 1½ cups alcohol-free witch hazel distillate
- 1 package round cotton pads

1 Combine yarrow, plantain, and witch hazel distillate in a pint-sized Mason jar and cover. Shake or stir to ensure that herbs are fully saturated.

2 Steep at least 2 weeks and up to 4 weeks, shaking the jar every other day. Add more witch hazel as needed to keep the herbs submerged.

3 After steeping is complete, strain the mixture into a bowl through a fine-mesh sieve or cheesecloth. Squeeze the spent herbs to extract as much liquid as possible. Store in a covered jar in the bathroom, near the cotton pads. Use within 6 months.

4 To use, soak a cotton pad in the herb-infused witch hazel and apply to the affected area after having a bowel movement or anytime you need relief. Make sure not to dip a used pad back into the witch hazel, as this will cause bacterial contamination.

remedy notes

For best results, combine this topical treatment with a high-fiber diet and regular consumption of Flaxseed Stool Softener (see recipe in this chapter) to keep your stools soft and easy to pass. Straining during bowel movements makes hemorrhoids much worse.

Chapter 7

EMOTIONAL BALANCE AND MENTAL HEALTH

The idea that it's possible to separate mind, body, and emotions is an illusion. You are whole. Taking care of your emotional and mental health is no different from taking care of any other part of your body. In fact, since stress is a major risk factor for most chronic diseases, taking care of your thoughts and emotions may turn out to be the best thing you can do for your physical well-being.

Being emotionally and mentally healthy isn't about feeling happy all the time. The goal is to cultivate a state of connection, flexibility, and relatedness that supports you in pursuing a life that's meaningful to you. Even unpleasant emotions serve a purpose; it's only when you get "stuck" in a state of chronic overwhelm, anger, fear, or sadness that you might need to turn to remedies for help. Herbs and natural remedies can relieve the emotional effects of stress, support your body through a grieving process, and make it easier to get a good night's sleep. They can help you to meet difficult moments with grace, resilience, and an ever-deepening connection to your heart. Here, you'll learn how to use natural remedies to bring yourself comfort, reduce the harmful effects of stress, and support the healthy functioning of your mind and emotions.

⊷ Calming Sesame Oil Massage ⊷

BENEFITS AND USES: *grounds your energy and calms your mind while moisturizing your skin*

AVOID: *if you're allergic to sesame oil*

YIELDS: 1 treatment

> 2 tablespoons unrefined sesame oil
> Hot water

1 Warm sesame oil by putting it into a 1-ounce plastic bottle and inserting the bottle into a larger cup or bowl of hot (but not boiling!) water.

2 Shower or bathe normally while the sesame oil warms up. Pat your skin dry with a towel. Then, starting with your toes and using strokes that move toward your heart, slowly massage the warm sesame oil into every inch of your skin.

3 Once you've worked as much oil into your skin as it can absorb, pat dry any excess oil that's left on the surface of your skin. Use an old towel for this since oil tends to stain fabric.

4 Repeat this practice a few times a week during the winter months. You can do this self-massage as often as every day if you're feeling dry, cold, stressed, or in need of grounding. This is an especially nice thing to do within 24 hours of air travel. (Hint: the less balanced you typically feel after air travel, the more likely it is that this remedy is a good match for your body type.)

Nighttime Nutmeg and Vanilla Hempseed Milk

BENEFITS AND USES: *soothes the mind and helps you to wind down before bed*

AVOID: *taking nutmeg in large doses. In amounts of more than a teaspoon or two, nutmeg is a hypnotic and a hallucinogen with unpleasant and potentially dangerous side effects.*

YIELDS: 2 servings

- ¼ cup hulled hemp seeds
- 2 cups water
- ½ teaspoon vanilla extract
- 1 medjool date, soaked in ½ cup water
- Scant ⅛ teaspoon sea salt
- ¼ teaspoon freshly grated nutmeg, divided

1 Combine all ingredients except nutmeg in a blender. Starting on low speed and slowly increasing to high speed, blend 1–2 minutes, until smooth and creamy.

2 If you want a perfectly smooth beverage, pour the milk through a fine-mesh strainer. To benefit from the fiber in the seeds and date, leave the beverage unstrained.

3 Warm the milk in the microwave or on the stovetop over medium heat until it's warm but not scalding hot. Divide evenly between two mugs and sprinkle ⅛ teaspoon nutmeg over each cup of warm milk. Then sip your way to relaxation and coziness.

✈ Relaxing Lavender Almond Latte ✈

BENEFITS AND USES: *calms the mind and the body*

AVOID: *N/A*

YIELDS: 1 serving

▸ **2 teaspoons dried lavender flowers**

▸ **½ cup hot water**

▸ **⅛ cup unsweetened almond milk, warmed**

▸ **2 teaspoons maple syrup**

1 Place lavender flowers in a paper tea filter or tea ball and place in a mug. Pour hot water over the lavender flowers. Cover and steep 7 minutes before removing tea filter.

2 Add warm almond milk and maple syrup to the strong lavender tea in the mug. Use a milk-frothing tool to whip up some foam on top, if you have one. Bring the mug with you to a cozy spot so you can fully relax as you sip.

 remedy notes

The relaxing properties of this preparation are gentle. If you have insomnia or anxiety, you may need to combine it with stronger remedies from this chapter to get results. More sedating herbs like skullcap and passionflower tend toward bitterness. If they help but you don't enjoy the taste, drink the bitter preparation first, then enjoy slowly sipping this yummy latte while its effects kick in.

Pick-Me-Up Peppermint Latte

BENEFITS AND USES: *helps you to feel awake and alert without caffeine or stimulants*

AVOID: *N/A*

YIELDS: 4 large servings

> 1 heaping cup dried peppermint leaf

> 4 cups boiling water

> 1⅓ cups soy milk, divided

---

1 Place peppermint in a clean Mason jar. Pour water over the peppermint, stirring if needed to make sure that all of the herb is fully saturated with water. Cover and let steep at least 15 minutes. Strain through a fine-mesh sieve to create a peppermint infusion. You can make one or more lattes immediately and/or store leftover peppermint infusion in a covered container in the refrigerator up to 48 hours.

2 For each hot latte, combine ¾ cup peppermint infusion with ⅓ cup warm soy milk in a large mug. If you prefer an iced drink, chill the peppermint infusion and use cold soy milk. Use the same proportions and procedure described in step 1, but pour the latte over ice in a glass before serving.

The strong aromatic quality of peppermint breaks up stagnation in the body and mind and seems to cut through mental fogginess and fatigue. I liken the effects to the "smelling salts" of old, strong fragrances used to revive people who were on the verge of swooning.

Cacao, Cayenne, and Cinnamon Hot Chocolate

BENEFITS AND USES: *provides comfort and lifts a low mood*

AVOID: *N/A*

YIELDS: 2 servings

- ½ cup full-fat canned coconut milk
- 1 cup unsweetened almond milk
- ¼ cup cacao powder
- ⅛ cup maple syrup
- ¼ teaspoon ground cinnamon
- ⅛ teaspoon ground ginger
- ⅛ teaspoon cayenne pepper
- ⅛ teaspoon sea salt

---

1 Add all ingredients to a high-speed blender. (Note: if the coconut milk appears solid after you open the can, it's because the cream has separated and risen to the top. To reverse the separation, pour the contents of the can into a heat-safe bowl, microwave on high 20 seconds, and whisk until cream is incorporated before measuring the amount you need for this recipe.)

2 Blend on low speed for a few seconds before slowly increasing to the highest speed. Continue to blend on high speed 90 seconds to ensure cacao powder dissolves fully in the liquid.

Cacao, Cayenne, and Cinnamon Hot Chocolate—continued

3 Warm the cocoa using either the microwave or stovetop. To micro-wave, divide cocoa evenly between two microwave-safe mugs. Place the first mug in the microwave and heat on high 1 minute, stir, then return to microwave another 30–60 seconds until hot. Repeat with the second mug. For the stovetop method, add all of the cocoa to a small, heavy-bottomed pot and warm over medium heat, stirring constantly until hot, about 5 minutes. Divide between two mugs and enjoy.

Long associated with the heart, cacao is a popular remedy for heartbreak and sadness. In this recipe, ginger, cinnamon, and cayenne stimulate circulation and keep the body's energy from becoming stagnant, while the fat from the coconut milk is ground-ing and comforting. If you're watching your cholesterol intake, you can substitute almond or soy milk for the full-fat coconut milk.

⤜ Goji Berry and Schisandra Elixir ⤛

BENEFITS AND USES: *lifts your mood and increases your resilience to all forms of stress*

AVOID: *N/A*

YIELDS: just over 1 cup; about 30 servings

- ▸ ½ **cup chopped dried goji berries**
- ▸ ½ **cup dried schisandra berries**
- ▸ **Slightly less than 1 cup brandy, divided**
- ▸ ½ **cup raw honey**

1 Combine goji and schisandra berries in a pint-sized Mason jar.

2 Pour brandy over berries in two stages. First, pour enough brandy into the jar to saturate and cover the berries (between ¼ and ½ cup). Then pour in another ½ cup or so, stopping when the level of the brandy is about 3" above the level of the berries.

3 Add honey and then gently stir with a knife or chopstick.

4 Label the jar and secure it with a lid. Let the elixir steep 6 weeks, shaking or stirring the jar a few times per week. After steeping, strain through a fine-mesh sieve into a wide-mouth Mason jar or liquid measuring cup, making sure to squeeze as much liquid from the spent berries as possible before discarding them.

5 To use, take up to ½ tablespoon elixir up to three times per day to support your mood and combat the effects of stress. You can take it directly from a spoon or mix with hot water to create an instant "tea."

 remedy notes

Goji berries are a nutritious, antioxidant-rich, mood-enhancing food that lends sweetness to this elixir. Schisandra berries help your body to become more resilient in the face of physical and emotional stress. They're believed to help stop the "leakage" of energy that I associate with common descriptions of the effects of chronic emotional stress, like feeling "drained" and "depleted."

Mood-Lifting Trail Mix

BENEFITS AND USES: *helps when you're feeling sad and run-down in the week before or during your period*

AVOID: *if you have headaches that are triggered by chocolate or caffeine*

YIELDS: 1½ cups (10 servings)

- ½ cup raw almonds
- ½ cup raw cacao nibs
- ½ cup dried goji berries

Add all ingredients to a large bowl. Stir together and enjoy!

remedy notes

Balancing the flavors of ingredients is a formulation technique for creating remedies with effects that are greater than the sum of their parts. This principle applies to trail mix too! Cacao nibs and goji berries both contain mood-enhancing compounds, but they balance each other in this formula because cacao is bitter and the goji berries are sweet and sour. The nourishing almonds mellow out the stronger actions of the cacao and goji berries with their neutral flavor.

❋ Sweet Dreams Syrup ❋

YIELDS: about 2 cups

- ¼ cup powdered ashwagandha root
- ¼ cup dried passionflower (above-ground parts)
- 4 cups water
- ½ cup dried chamomile flowers
- 1 teaspoon freshly grated nutmeg
- ½ cup blackstrap molasses
- ½ cup raw honey

1 Add ashwagandha root, passionflower, and water to a medium pot and bring to a boil. As soon as the mixture reaches a full boil, reduce heat and simmer gently for 10 minutes.

2 Add chamomile flowers and nutmeg. Partially cover the pot with a lid and continue to simmer until the water is reduced to half its original volume, about 10–15 more minutes. (You can measure the volume of the liquid by inserting a chopstick into the pot before it reaches its initial boil so that the water level "marks" the chopstick. When you think you're getting close to the halfway point, insert the same chopstick to gauge how much the liquid has reduced.)

3 Once the liquid has reduced by half, strain the decoction through a fine-mesh sieve into a quart-sized Mason jar. (Discard the dregs containing the remains of the powdered ashwagandha.) Add molasses and honey to the Mason jar and stir until all ingredients are combined. Store syrup in the refrigerator up to 1 month.

Sweet Dreams Syrup—continued

4 To use the syrup for sleep support, take 1 tablespoon around dinner-time and another 1 tablespoon about an hour before bed. You may safely combine this nourishing remedy with a sedative remedy like skullcap or passionflower tincture if you need extra help falling asleep.

remedy notes

Blackstrap molasses has a high iron content that helps prevent iron-deficiency anemia, a common cause of bad dreams and insomnia. But if you're not anemic and you don't like the taste of molasses, feel free to replace with honey. *Note: do not combine this remedy with antianxiety medication, sedatives, or hypnotics unless advised to do so by your healthcare provider.*

✦ Ashwagandha Coconut Milk ✦

BENEFITS AND USES: *counteracts stress when you're both tired and wired or if you have slightly low thyroid function*

AVOID: *if you have an overactive thyroid*

YIELDS: 1 serving

- ¾ cup water
- ¼ cup full-fat canned coconut milk
- 1 teaspoon powdered ashwagandha (*Withania somnifera*) root
- 1 teaspoon raw honey
- ¼ teaspoon freshly grated nutmeg

1 Combine water, coconut milk, and ashwagandha powder in a small pot with a wide diameter. Bring to a boil and then reduce heat to a simmer. Simmer gently, uncovered, until reduced by half, about 10–15 minutes. (The wider your pot, the less time it will take to reduce the liquid.)

2 Pour into a mug, add honey, and stir gently until honey is incorporated. Top with freshly grated nutmeg. Drink after dinner to encourage sound sleep.

 remedy notes

Most adaptogens (herbs that improve resilience to physical and emotional stress) are stimulating and can interfere with sleep if you take them too close to bedtime. Ashwagandha is special; it's the only adaptogen that's also sleep promoting. This makes it the perfect herb for people who are so tired and depleted that it's as if they don't even have the energy to fall asleep. (This sounds strange—until you experience it!)

Lavender and Chamomile
Anxiety Relief Tea

BENEFITS AND USES: *helps with anxiety accompanied by abdominal tension, loss of appetite, or upset stomach*

AVOID: *N/A*

YIELDS: 1 cup

> 2 teaspoons dried lavender flowers
> 2 teaspoons dried chamomile flowers
> 1 cup hot water

1 Measure the lavender and chamomile flowers into a small bowl and toss gently to combine. Add the dried herbs to a paper tea filter, tea strainer, or tea ball and place inside a mug or teacup.

2 Pour hot water over the herbs, cover with a saucer, and let steep 10 minutes before serving. Sip this tea slowly, breathing in the aroma of the herbs and noticing the effects that they have on your mind and body. Breathing, tasting, and noticing how you feel are part of the medicine.

remedy notes

If you don't want to blend your own loose herbs, Traditional Medicinals (www.traditionalmedicinals.com) makes a lovely Chamomile with Lavender tea that's prepackaged into tea bags. If you use a commercially prepared tea, remember to use two tea bags per cup of tea when you desire a medicinal effect. A single bag is perfectly fine if you just want a nice hot beverage.

⤙ Holiday Happiness Syrup ⤚

BENEFITS AND USES: *relieves and prevents all manner of holiday stress*

AVOID: *if you're taking blood thinners or blood pressure medication (ask your doctor before using this formula)*

YIELDS: about 6 cups

- ½ cup dried schisandra berries
- Heaping ½ cup dried hawthorn berries
- ¼ cup dried rose hips
- ¼ cup green cardamom pods
- 5 whole cloves
- 1 cinnamon stick
- 3" knob fresh ginger root, peeled and sliced
- 12 cups water
- 1½ cups sugar

1 Add all ingredients except sugar to a large pot and bring to a boil. As soon as the liquid reaches a full boil, turn down the heat to a simmer. Allow to simmer about 30–40 minutes, until the volume of the liquid is reduced by half. (The wider the diameter of your pot, the faster the liquid will reduce.) When it's ready, the liquid will have thickened slightly and turned a deep garnet color.

Holiday Happiness Syrup—continued

2   Strain the decoction through a fine-mesh sieve into a liquid measuring cup large enough to hold at least 6 cups and discard solids. Measure the amount of liquid and divide that measurement in half to determine the perfect amount of sugar to add. This should be approximately 1½ cups, but it's worthwhile to measure your decoction since the exact volume is likely to vary each time you make this recipe. The sugar works as a preservative, so don't reduce the amount. Add the sugar and stir until completely dissolved. (You can return the liquid to the pot and warm over low heat for a few minutes if you're having trouble getting the sugar to dissolve.) Store syrup in a covered jar in the refrigerator and use within 1 month.

3   There are lots of ways to use this syrup. You can take it once or twice per day as a preventive tonic to bolster yourself during times of stress. (Dose: 1 teaspoon for children ages 6–12; 1 tablespoon for adults and children over 12.) You can also use it to sweeten other herbal teas, or add 1 tablespoon to a glass and slowly pour in 1 cup seltzer to create an Italian soda.

remedy notes

Schisandra berries are prized in Chinese medicine for their ability to settle the spirit, prevent the leakage of vital energy, and strengthen the body's resilience to stress. Hawthorn berries prevent and treat "food stagnation" (a familiar feeling for many people after overindulging on Thanksgiving!). Cardamom, clove, cinnamon, and ginger help to warm up the formula and further support good digestion. They also make the house smell heavenly while the syrup is cooking!

Rosemary Lemon "Remembrance" Tea

BENEFITS AND USES: *increases your memory and focus*

AVOID: *N/A*

YIELDS: 4 servings

- **4 sprigs fresh rosemary**
- **Juice of 1 organic lemon, plus ¼ of the peel**
- **6 cups water**
- **1 heaping tablespoon sugar**

---

1 Add rosemary, lemon peel, and water to a medium pot. Bring to a boil and then reduce heat to a simmer and partially cover. Simmer gently for 20–30 minutes.

2 Add the lemon juice and sugar.

3 To serve, place a small strainer over your mug. Ladle 1 cup tea into the mug through the strainer. You can either prepare three more mugs to share with others or strain the leftover tea into a Mason jar and store in the fridge up to 48 hours to enjoy later. Savor the refreshing aroma as you sip the tea. The enlivening fragrance is an important part of this remedy, so make sure to tune into your senses and really breathe it in.

remedy notes

This is the perfect remedy for late-night study sessions or work meetings when you need some help focusing but don't want to drink anything caffeinated that could interfere with your sleep. After all, good sleep is vital for healthy memory and enhances learning. When it's hot outside, chill and serve this recipe over ice as a lemonade for similar benefits.

✦ Rose Oil Heart-Opening Ritual ✦

BENEFITS AND USES: *awakens compassion for yourself and others*

AVOID: *N/A*

YIELDS: 1 treatment

➤ **4–5 drops 10 percent dilution rose absolute in carrier oil**

1 Take a few deep breaths and then massage a few drops of the diluted rose absolute oil into the area around your heart. As you do this, feel the sensations at the center of your chest. Feel your heartbeat with the palm of your hand. Then see if you can drop your awareness deep into the area around your heart so that you can feel your heart beating inside your chest.

2 Continuing to sense the area around your heart, imagine that you're breathing directly into and out of the space around your heart. I often invite my clients to imagine that there are beautiful French doors at the front and back of the chest. Visualize those doors (close your eyes if that helps!) and imagine that you could swing them wide open to allow your breath to flow through.

3 Allow yourself to luxuriate in the fragrance of roses as you continue to feel your heart and breathe into the center of your chest. To complete the practice, call up a memory or image of something that brings you a feeling of true gratitude. This could be a beautiful scene in nature, a favorite meal, or someone in your life (person or animal) who you can trust. Feel the emotion of gratitude as you continue to breathe into your heart. When you're ready to conclude the exercise, open your eyes if you closed them before and say "thank you" either out loud or silently to yourself.

Neroli Antidepressant Anointing Oil

BENEFITS AND USES: *provides extra support during times of sadness, grief, and depression*

AVOID: *if you're allergic to citrus*

YIELDS: about 15 applications

- ¾ tablespoon unrefined sesame oil
- 1½ teaspoons 10 percent dilution neroli essential oil in carrier oil

1 Combine sesame oil and diluted neroli essential oil in a 1-ounce bottle fitted with a dropper. Close the bottle and shake well.

2 To use, apply 3–4 dropperfuls to your body before getting dressed in the morning and massage into your skin until absorbed. As you apply the oil, breathe in the comforting fragrance and imagine that you're applying a layer of loving protection that will stay with you through-out the day. Adding this imagery to the ritual of applying the oil will engage your mind in the healing process and enhance your results.

3 If you don't have time to apply this oil to your whole body, or if you need a little extra support during the day, massage a drop or two of oil into your pulse points or over your heart.

remedy notes

Sadness, grief, and depression can sometimes be accompanied by muscle aches, pain, and fatigue. If you tend to experience bodily symptoms like these during times of sadness, you can sub-stitute St. John's Wort–infused oil for the sesame oil. St. John's Wort has a great affinity for the nervous system, and applying it topi-cally can help you receive the pain-relieving benefits without the risk of herb/drug interactions that comes from taking it internally. (Note: this remedy is not designed to replace appropriate medical and psychological treatment.)

Skullcap and Kuzu Root Tension Reliever

BENEFITS AND USES: *unwinds tense neck, shoulder, and jaw muscles*

AVOID: *using with medications that lower blood pressure or have anxiety-relieving, muscle-relaxant, and/or sedative properties*

YIELDS: 1 cup

> 1 tablespoon dried skullcap (*Scutellaria lateriflora*)
> 1 cup hot water
> 2 teaspoons kuzu root powder

1 Place skullcap in a paper tea filter, tea ball, or small tea strainer basket and add to a mug. Pour ¾ cup of the hot water into the mug and let the tea steep 10 minutes before removing the skullcap.

2 Add kuzu root powder to the mug. Use a small whisk to stir until kuzu is dissolved, about 1–2 minutes, and drink immediately.

remedy notes

Skullcap is a bitter-tasting plant in the mint family that's particularly helpful when there's a feeling of anger or frustration lurking right behind your stress. This is the remedy to turn to when you're wound too tight and feel like you might explode. For even better results, drink this tea before soaking in the Dead Sea Salt Bath for Stress Relief (see recipe in this chapter).

⤝ Dead Sea Salt Bath for Stress Relief ⤞

BENEFITS AND USES: *relieves stress that's accompanied by tight neck, shoulder, and upper back muscles*

AVOID: *if you have high blood pressure, are pregnant, or have open wounds or diabetic ulcers*

YIELDS: 1 treatment

- **2 cups Epsom salt**
- **1 cup Dead Sea salt**
- **20 drops Roman chamomile essential oil**
- **5 drops geranium essential oil**
- **5 drops nutmeg essential oil**
- **1 hand towel**

1 Draw a hot (but not scalding) bath and dissolve the Epsom salt and Dead Sea salt in the hot water. Add essential oils, swish the water around with your hand, and then get into the tub.

2 Make a compress by soaking the hand towel in the hot bath water and draping it around your neck and shoulders. Once it gets cool, dip it back into the bath and squeeze it a few times so that it heats up and absorbs fresh bath water. Continue to apply the compress to your neck and shoulders for as long as it feels good, up to 30 minutes.

 remedy notes

The Epsom salt encourages muscle relaxation, while the Dead Sea salt pampers your skin. Roman chamomile's muscle-relaxant properties work even better with the support of geranium to lift your mood and nutmeg to relax your mind. You can also try sipping either the Lavender and Chamomile Anxiety Relief Tea or the Skullcap and Kuzu Root Tension Reliever (see recipes in this chapter) to complement this bath perfectly.

⤙ Simple Sunrise Medicine ⤚

BENEFITS AND USES: *supports daytime energy, focus, and mood while promoting restful sleep at night. It's especially helpful for mild depression accompanying hypothyroidism.*

AVOID: *N/A*

YIELDS: 1 day of improved mood and energy

➤ **The sun**

1 Go outside for at least 20 minutes as close to sunrise as you can manage. This works on sunny and cloudy days alike, but it doesn't work very well if you watch the sunrise through windows. (Being in your car probably provides enough light exposure, though.) If you're really not a morning person, it's okay to go back to bed after you spend your time outside.

2 If getting up in time for sunrise feels like an impossible task, start slow. Go outside for 20 minutes as soon as you wake up. Do this for a week or so. Then try getting up 30–90 minutes earlier, going outside for light exposure, and giving yourself permission to go back to bed if you want to. The closer you get to sunrise, the more you'll notice the benefits.

remedy notes

This remedy is one of my favorites because it's completely free from side effects, costs nothing, and has a profound effect on your body and mind. It works by resetting your circadian rhythm, which affects the hormone levels and neurochemicals involved in everything from your mood, sleep, and stress response to your metabolism and reproductive cycles. In fact, morning sunlight exposure is one of the best natural remedies for any kind of hormonal imbalance and has been a key part of the success I've had with clients who have impaired thyroid function, sleep disorders, or infertility.

St. John's Wort for Seasonal Mood Support

BENEFITS AND USES: *helps with mild to moderate depression, especially when the depression is a component of seasonal affective disorder (SAD)*

AVOID: *if you take prescription medications of any kind or have bipolar disorder, major depressive disorder, postpartum depression, or thoughts of harming yourself or others*

YIELDS: approximately 3 weeks of mood support

› 1 (1-ounce) bottle St. John's Wort (*Hypericum perforatum*) tincture
› ⅛ cup water per dose

1 Determine your dose. Adult women weighing less than 130 pounds should start with ¼ teaspoon twice per day, those weighing between 130 and 160 pounds can start with ½ teaspoon twice per day, and those weighing 175 pounds or more can start with ¾ teaspoon twice per day. No matter your size, you can slowly increase to as much as 1½ teaspoons per dose (up to 3 teaspoons total per day), if needed.

2 Measure the appropriate dose of tincture into a small amount of water (at least ⅛ cup, but use more if you prefer) and drink. It's okay to take with food or by itself. Start with the lower dosing range split into a morning and evening dose if you can remember to take it twice per day. (If not, it's okay to take the full dose in the morning.)

3 Notice how you feel after 1 week. If you haven't noticed much improvement, increase to the mid-range dose and observe yourself for another week. If there's still no improvement, increase to the full dose and consider reaching out for additional support just in case you don't get relief from the full dose after another week.

Uplifting Lemon Balm Anointing Oil

BENEFITS AND USES: *lifts your mood, energizes body and mind, and maybe even puts a smile on your face in the midst of seasonal depression*

AVOID: *if you're allergic to any members of the mint family or are pregnant*

YIELDS: 1 (1-ounce) bottle (approximately 30 applications)

- ¾ tablespoon jojoba oil
- 1½ teaspoons 10 percent dilution lemon balm essential oil

1 Combine oils in a 1-ounce bottle fitted with a dropper. Shake well.

2 To use, apply a dropperful of oil to your body, or use for inhalation anytime your spirits need a lift. For an instant inhalation, rub 5 drops of the anointing oil between your palms. Then cover your nose and mouth with your hands and breathe deeply 30–90 seconds. The warmth of your palms releases the oils' full fragrance. I think of this practice as a way to "put on your own oxygen mask first" during times of stress and sadness.

 remedy notes

Since lemon balm (*Melissa officinalis*) essential oil is expensive to produce, manufacturers usually bottle it as a 10 percent dilution. Dilution doesn't affect the quality; it just makes the product more affordable and slightly changes how you'll use it. It's safe to put a drop of 10 percent essential oil dilution directly on your pulse points, but avoid using it in a diffuser or in water-based recipes.

Powerful Passionflower and Skullcap Tea

BENEFITS AND USES: *relieves significant anxiety and sedates the nervous system*

AVOID: *if pregnant or breastfeeding or if taking opioids or medications for anxiety, blood pressure, seizures, or sleep. Do not use before driving or operating heavy machinery.*

YIELDS: 2 servings

> 1 heaping tablespoon dried passionflower
> 1 heaping tablespoon dried skullcap
> 1 tablespoon dried catnip
> 1 tablespoon dried chamomile flowers
> 2 cups hot water

1 Add herbs to a French press or a teapot with a built-in strainer. (If you don't have a French press or a teapot, you can use a Mason jar and strain the mixture through a fine-mesh sieve before drinking.)

2 Pour hot water over herbs and cover. Let the tea steep 15–20 minutes and then strain and drink. You should feel some relief within 10 minutes of finishing the tea. If not, drink the second cup. If you don't notice a marked reduction in anxiety after drinking this tea, you need either a different remedy or a higher dose. It's safe to drink multiple batches, if needed.

remedy notes

Anxiety is a physical state, not just a set of worried thoughts. This blend calms the central nervous system and helps to dial down the physical side of your anxiety so that you can rein in your thoughts more easily. While these herbs calm significant anxiety, they do not carry risks of overdose or addiction like benzodiazepines. You can use this formula regularly without risk of physical dependence, but if you're having frequent anxiety, the best thing to do is to seek out a qualified therapist.

Chapter 8

FITNESS AND FLEXIBILITY

Physical fitness is measured across multiple dimensions: cardio-vascular health, strength, balance, flexibility, and metabolic health. The more fitness you have in each area, the healthier you are. The best way to increase your fitness is by balancing good stressors (e.g., physical exercise) with excellent nutrition and periods of rest. It's during the recovery period that your body rebuilds itself and becomes stronger. If you want to improve your fitness, you have to strike a balance between challenging yourself and giving your body what it needs to rebuild. While this chapter can't do your workouts for you, it *is* full of remedies that will supply your body with nutrients, antioxidants, and beneficial plant compounds to help you get the most out of your recovery periods.

While this balance of rest and exercise is crucial for cardiovascular health, the food you eat matters too. Here, you'll find recipes that make it easy and delicious to include heart-healthy herbs like garlic and hawthorn in your diet to reduce the risk of heart disease. And since injuries and accidents happen, this chapter also includes remedies like muscle rubs and liniments that you'll want to have on hand for those times when your active lifestyle results in bumps and bruises.

⇻ Citrus and Sea Salt ⇺ Electrolyte Replenisher

BENEFITS AND USES: *hydrates during long workouts or on very hot days*

AVOID: *N/A*

YIELDS: 2 servings

› **1 cup freshly squeezed lemon juice**

› **⅛ teaspoon fine-grain sea salt**

› **1 tablespoon grade B maple syrup**

› **4 cups water**

Stir all ingredients together in a quart-sized Mason jar. Pour into individual glasses or water bottles to serve or to take with you to hydrate after exertion.

remedy notes

You don't need fancy sports drinks to rehydrate yourself during heavy physical exertion or after fluid loss. This homemade formula works just as well! If needed, you can double, triple, or quadruple the recipe to fill a large water bottle before a long training session, day of hiking, or other event where you'll need to replace electrolytes.

⇢ Turmeric Paste ⇠

BENEFITS AND USES: *protects cells from damage and reduces inflammation*

AVOID: *if turmeric is a migraine trigger for you; using with blood thinners, proton pump inhibitors, or other medications that reduce stomach acid production*

YIELDS: about ⅓ cup

- ¼ cup turmeric powder
- ½ teaspoon ground black pepper
- ½ cup water

1   Combine all ingredients in a small pot and heat over medium-low heat. Whisk or stir until the mixture forms a very thick paste, about 5 minutes.

2   Transfer turmeric paste to a glass jar and store in the refrigerator up to 2 weeks.

3   To use, remove from fridge and eat ¼ teaspoon up to twice per day, or incorporate into another recipe in this book.

remedy notes

Combining turmeric with black pepper helps to make some of its most beneficial compounds more bioavailable—so don't skip the pepper! If the taste is too intense for you, mix your turmeric paste with ¼ teaspoon honey before consuming or try one of the many recipes in this book that use turmeric paste.

❧ Eleuthero Miso Soup ❧

BENEFITS AND USES: *enhances recovery, supports more effective athletic training, and increases your resilience to stress*

AVOID: *if you're taking blood thinners*

YIELDS: 4 servings

> 1 tablespoon olive oil
> 2 cloves garlic, smashed and peeled
> ⅛ teaspoon ground turmeric
> ¼ cup dried eleuthero (*Eleutherococcus senticosus*) root
> 3" knob fresh ginger root, peeled and sliced
> 6 cups water
> 8 ounces firm silken tofu, cubed
> 4 scant tablespoons miso paste, divided
> 1 small bunch scallions, chopped

1 Add olive oil, garlic, and turmeric to a small pot and warm over medium heat until garlic is fragrant, about 3–4 minutes. Meanwhile, lay eleuthero root onto a piece of cheesecloth and tie into a loose bundle. (This will save you the step of having to strain the broth later, but if you don't have any cheesecloth, it's okay to skip this step and simply strain the broth after step 3.)

2 Add sliced ginger root to the pot and cook 1–2 minutes, stirring constantly. Add water to the pot along with the eleuthero root bundle. Cover the pot and bring to a rolling boil. Then turn down the heat to a simmer and partially uncover the pot. Allow broth to simmer until the total volume is reduced by ¼, about 20 minutes.

3 Remove the eleuthero bundle, add tofu to the hot broth, and cook another 3–4 minutes, until tofu is warmed through.

Eleuthero Miso Soup—continued

4 To serve, spoon 1 scant tablespoon miso paste into each serving bowl. Add a ladleful of hot (but not boiling) broth to each bowl and use the back of a spoon to help the miso paste dissolve evenly into the broth. Add broth until each bowl is full (approximately 1 cup per bowl) and garnish each bowl with a heaping tablespoon of the chopped fresh scallions.

If you have a soy allergy, you can use chickpea or azuki bean miso. You can omit the tofu and serve this as a broth, or substitute "tofu" made from chickpea flour. This recipe would also work well made with astragalus root instead of or in addition to the eleuthero for people who need more immune system support.

⤜ Golden Milk ⤛

BENEFITS AND USES: *supports vitality and reduces inflammation*

AVOID: *if turmeric is a migraine trigger for you or if you're taking blood thinners, proton pump inhibitors, or other medications that reduce stomach acid production*

YIELDS: 1 serving

- ▸ **1 cup unsweetened almond milk**
- ▸ **½ teaspoon Turmeric Paste (see recipe in this chapter)**

1 Combine all ingredients in a small pot. Whisk together over medium heat until warmed through and well combined, about 3 minutes.

2 Pour into your favorite cup and sip to your heart's (and tummy's and joints') content!

remedy notes

If you don't fancy the taste of golden milk right away, you can add a teaspoon of maple syrup, honey, or another sweetener. Turmeric stains fabric, so be careful not to get it on your favorite clothing or fancy dish towel. If you accidentally spill some on your counter, clean it up right away so it won't leave a mark.

☀ Garlic Gremolata ☀

BENEFITS AND USES: *helps you get the heart-healthy benefits of raw garlic*

AVOID: *if you have FODMAP-sensitive IBS and garlic is a trigger for you*

YIELDS: 1 scant cup (enough to garnish a dish that serves 4–6 people)

- 1 small bunch fresh flat-leaf parsley, finely chopped (about 1 cup, loosely packed)
- 1 clove garlic, peeled
- 1 organic lemon

1 Add parsley leaves to a serving dish and then grate the garlic clove over the parsley. Zest lemon over parsley and garlic. Toss to combine. The mixture will be dry and easy to sprinkle.

2 To use, sprinkle over food while the food is still warm. Gremolata is best when consumed right away, but you can store leftovers in a covered container in the fridge and use within 24 hours.

remedy notes

Gremolata is a perfect illustration of the way that herbs with different flavors come together to form something greater than the sum of the parts. Here, the cooling, aromatic parsley balances the hot, pungent garlic. Gremolata is delicious when used to top steamed or roasted vegetables, pasta dishes, soups, or roasted potatoes.

✈ Triple Adaptogen Tincture ✈

BENEFITS AND USES: *builds your resilience to physical and emotional stress*

AVOID: *if you're pregnant or taking blood thinners, immunosuppressants, corticosteroids, antipsychotic or anti-seizure medications*

YIELDS: about 1½ cups

- ⅓ cup dried eleuthero (*Eleutherococcus senticosus*) root
- ⅓ cup dried ashwagandha root (or ¼ cup powdered)
- ⅓ cup dried schisandra berries
- ¼ cup boiling water
- ½ tablespoon dried licorice root
- 3" knob fresh ginger root, peeled and finely chopped
- 3½ cups brandy, divided
- ⅛ cup water (or more as desired) per dose

---

1 Add eleuthero, ashwagandha, and schisandra berries to a quart-sized Mason jar.

2 Pour hot water over herbs and stir once or twice with a knife to saturate evenly. Let stand 5 minutes.

3 Add the licorice root and chopped ginger to the Mason jar. Cover herb mixture with 3 cups brandy. Secure the jar with a lid and attach a label that includes the name of the remedy, the ingredients, and the date. Set aside overnight.

4 The next day, check the jar. If the herbs have swollen to take up more than half of the volume of the jar, add up to another ½ cup or so of brandy. Let tincture macerate at least 3 weeks and up to 6 weeks. Shake the jar a few times per week.

Triple Adaptogen Tincture—continued

5 When you're ready to bottle the finished tincture, strain through a fine-mesh sieve lined with cheesecloth. Make sure to squeeze as much alcohol from the spent herbs as possible! Bottle and label the finished tincture and store away from direct sunlight and extreme temperatures. Your tincture will be safe to use for up to 5 years, though it will start to slowly lose potency after 1 year or so.

6 To use, take ½ teaspoon in water (at least ⅛ cup or up to a full glass, depending on your preference) every morning.

Adaptogenic herbs are named after their ability to help the body adapt to stress. Russian scientists searching for ways to support elite cosmonauts and Olympians were among the first to document that adaptogens are safe, that they are beneficial to multiple body systems, and that they increase resilience to physical and emotional stress. This formula features three famous adaptogens—eleuthero (formerly "Siberian ginseng"), ashwagandha, and schisandra berries—with ginger and licorice to harmonize the formula.

Better Than Garlic Butter

BENEFITS AND USES: *helps you get the heart-healthy benefits of raw garlic without eating it in its raw state*

AVOID: *if you have gastroesophageal reflux disease (GERD) or FODMAP-sensitive IBS and garlic is a trigger for you*

YIELDS: about ½ cup

- 1 whole head garlic
- ¼ cup extra-virgin olive oil
- ¼ teaspoon sea salt

1 Preheat oven to 325°F.

2 Peel and finely chop the garlic and let stand 5 minutes. The action of chopping the garlic and waiting for a few minutes releases the beneficial compounds so that they'll be bioavailable after roasting.

3 Add chopped garlic and olive oil to a medium baking dish. Sprinkle with sea salt.

4 Put baking dish in the oven and set the timer for 10 minutes. Since the garlic is chopped finely, it will burn if left unattended or if the oven gets too hot. To prevent this, check on it after 7 minutes. If any garlic is starting to brown, remove the dish from the oven immediately and stir before leaving it alone to cool. If the garlic is still a pale whitish yellow with no browning, stir once and continue to roast for the 3 remaining minutes.

5 Remove from oven and allow to cool. Store in a glass jar in the fridge up to 3 weeks. Consume 2 teaspoons daily for cardiovascular and anti-cancer benefits. Use doses as high as 3–4 tablespoons per day (as much as you can tolerate!) when fighting an infection.

 remedy notes

This remedy is tastiest when incorporated into food. Try stirring it into canned soup or store-bought hummus or add it to marinades for tofu, tempeh, or meat. Use it to top a baked potato, spread on toast, or use to make quick garlicky greens!

Muscle-Loving Omega-3 Brownie Bites

BENEFITS AND USES: *nourishes your body with omega-3 fatty acids, magnesium, and fiber*

AVOID: *if you're sensitive to sweets or chocolate*

YIELDS: 16–24 brownie bites

- 1¼ cups raw unsalted walnut halves or pieces
- ¼ cup hulled hemp seeds (or substitute another ¼ cup walnuts)
- ½ cup cacao powder
- ⅛ teaspoon sea salt
- 1 cup pitted medjool dates

1 Place walnuts, hemp seeds, cacao, and salt into a food processor. Pulse the mixture a few times until the walnuts are finely chopped, but don't overmix. A little bit of chunkiness is good.

2 Add pitted dates and pulse the food processor until the mixture is combined, about 1–2 minutes of pulsing. It's done when there are no large chunks and the mixture resembles sticky brownie crumbs.

3 If serving right away, choose a serving dish to hold the brownie bites. Otherwise, line a tin or plastic food storage container with parchment or wax paper. Shape the dough into brownie bites by taking approximately 1 tablespoon of the mixture and rolling it between clean hands until it resembles a small ball or truffle. Place on serving dish or inside the lined tin. Store in the refrigerator up to 4 days and serve at room temperature or chilled, according to your preference.

remedy notes

These brownie bites are a great alternative to less wholesome treats if you have chocolate cravings during PMS. Cacao supplies magnesium (which helps to relax muscles) and compounds that trigger both the pain-relief and happiness circuits in the brain. Chocolate is actually good medicine for PMS when it's combined with omega-3 fats and free from refined sugar and dairy!

⤜ Post-Workout Recovery Smoothie ⤛

BENEFITS AND USES: *replenishes your body after a workout*

AVOID: *if you're taking blood thinners or are allergic to soy*

YIELDS: 1 serving as a meal replacement; 2 servings as a snack

- ½ cup fresh or frozen strawberries
- ½ cup fresh or frozen raspberries
- ¾ cup frozen banana slices
- 1 cup fresh baby spinach leaves
- 2 tablespoons hulled hemp seeds
- 1 tablespoon chia seeds
- 1 tablespoon dried goji berries
- 1 medjool date, pitted
- 1½ cups soy milk
- 1" piece fresh ginger root, peeled

1 Add all ingredients to a blender and puree until smooth. If you like a thinner smoothie, add water until you reach the desired consistency.

2 Store leftovers in the fridge up to 24 hours.

remedy notes

The window of time after a workout is a nutritional opportunity that athletes and body builders don't want to miss. This smoothie has hemp seeds and soy milk to provide the protein muscles crave after being worked hard, along with healthy carbohydrates to replenish glycogen stores. If you're allergic to soy, replace the soy milk with a combination of almond milk and a scoop of rice or hemp protein powder.

⇥ Cholesterol-Lowering Overnight Oats ⇤

BENEFITS AND USES: *reduces anxiety and lowers cholesterol*

AVOID: *if you're gluten intolerant or allergic to soy*

YIELDS: 5 servings

OATMEAL:
- 1⅔ cups old-fashioned rolled oats
- 1½ teaspoons ground cinnamon
- ¼ cup plus 1 tablespoon chia seeds
- ¼ teaspoon sea salt
- ¼ cup plus 1 tablespoon almond butter
- 2 tablespoons vanilla extract
- 2½ cups soy milk

BANANA WALNUT TOPPING (PER SERVING):
- ½ banana, mashed
- ¼ cup toasted walnuts

ANTIOXIDANT TOPPING (PER SERVING):
- ½ cup blueberries
- ½ cup strawberries, sliced

HEART-LOVERS BREAKFAST TOPPING (PER SERVING):
- 2 tablespoons Hawthorn Goji Berry Jam (see recipe in this chapter)
- ¼ cup hulled hemp seeds

1 *For oatmeal:* Mix together oats, cinnamon, chia seeds, and salt in a large bowl or Mason jar. Add almond butter, vanilla extract, and soy milk and stir to combine. Let mixture sit in the fridge overnight before serving.

2 *For toppings:* To serve, scoop out ¾ cup oatmeal and top with one of the listed combinations.

Hawthorn Goji Berry Jam

BENEFITS AND USES: *supports heart health and a good mood*

AVOID: *overeating this recipe since it contains a relatively high amount of sugar*

YIELDS: about 1 cup

- ½ cup dried hawthorn berries
- 2 cups water
- ½ cup balsamic vinegar
- ½ cup granulated cane sugar
- 1 tablespoon arrowroot powder
- ½ cup (packed) roughly chopped dried goji berries

1 Combine hawthorn berries, water, vinegar, and sugar in a medium pot and bring to a boil. Reduce heat to low and simmer 20 minutes or until slightly thickened and reduced by about ⅓.

2 Remove the pot from the heat. Strain the mixture through a fine-mesh sieve into a heat-safe bowl, making sure to squeeze as much liquid from the spent berries as possible. Use a paper towel to wipe any remaining solids from the pot.

3 Return the liquid to the pot and whisk in the arrowroot powder. Simmer over low heat 2 more minutes or until thickened. The syrup is ready when it coats the back of a spoon.

4 Stir goji berries into the syrup and stir to combine. Transfer to a heat-safe jar and refrigerate. The jam will keep in the fridge about 1 month.

remedy notes

Hawthorn and goji berries confer the greatest benefits when they're a consistent part of your diet. Cooking them into a jam makes it possible to get a serving of these herbs without having to resort to a supplement or another cup of tea. Even though there's sugar in the recipe, this jam has benefits that you won't find in store-bought jams and jellies.

✈ The Ultimate Epsom Salt Bath ✈

BENEFITS AND USES: *encourages deep relaxation, relieves muscle soreness, and helps your body to unwind*

AVOID: *if you're pregnant or if you have uncontrolled high blood pressure*

YIELDS: 1 bath

➤ **2 cups Epsom salt**

➤ **1 cup Dead Sea salt**

➤ **5 drops lavender essential oil**

➤ **7 drops Roman chamomile essential oil**

➤ **5 drops German chamomile essential oil**

1 Draw a hot, but not scalding, bath and dissolve the Epsom salt and Dead Sea salt in the hot water. Add essential oils and swish the water around with your hand before getting into the tub.

2 Soak for 20–30 minutes and relax.

3 For best results, pat your skin dry with a towel and follow with Peppermint White Chocolate Body Butter (see Chapter 4) or Calming Sesame Oil Massage (see Chapter 7).

remedy notes

Epsom salt is a form of magnesium, a vital mineral for muscle relaxation, cardiac health, and emotional balance. Lavender calms the mind, Roman chamomile relieves muscle tension, and German chamomile imparts its anti-inflammatory powers to soothe your skin. If you can't take a hot bath, consider using this as a foot soak instead to get similar benefits. For a foot soak, use half the amount of each ingredient.

→ Ginger and Yarrow Deep Tissue Oil ↞

BENEFITS AND USES: *relieves deep muscle soreness from soft tissue injuries, overexertion, or delayed-onset muscle soreness after working out*

AVOID: *using internally or on broken skin*

YIELDS: a little more than 1½ cups

- ½ cup dried yarrow
- 6" knob fresh ginger root, peeled and sliced
- 3 fresh habanero peppers (including the seeds), split in half lengthwise
- 2 cups jojoba oil
- 5 drops rosemary essential oil
- 5 drops clary sage essential oil
- 5 drops geranium essential oil
- 5 drops Roman chamomile essential oil

1 Combine yarrow, ginger, habanero peppers, and jojoba oil in a quart-sized Mason jar and stir to combine. Cover the jar with a lid and label with the date and the ingredients. Allow to infuse in a sunny spot for 4 weeks, shaking the jar a few times per week. If you don't want to wait, you can infuse the oil by adding the first four ingredients to a double boiler, yogurt maker, or dehydrator and infuse using very gentle heat for a few hours until the oil is fragrant.

2 After the mixture is finished infusing, strain through a fine-mesh sieve lined with cheesecloth into a clean quart-sized Mason jar or glass liquid measuring cup. Add the essential oils to the infused oil and stir to combine. To store, you can return the oil to its original Mason jar (after wiping it out with a paper towel to remove any stray herbs) or pour into smaller bottles. Store at cool room temperature and use within 6 months.

Ginger and Yarrow Deep Tissue Oil—continued

3 To use, massage a small amount of oil into affected areas. If desired, apply heat to the affected muscles after applying the oil to help the oil to penetrate more deeply.

Since this oil increases circulation, your skin may become red and/or warm after application. This therapeutic effect isn't a cause for concern, but it's the reason why you need to keep this oil away from delicate mucus membranes. After applying, make sure not to touch your eyes, nose, mouth, or genitals until after you wash your hands. If you have sensitive skin, test on a small area before using more liberally.

Muscle Release Liniment

BENEFITS AND USES: *releases muscle tension and emotional stress that's being held in your muscles*

AVOID: *using internally*

YIELDS: about 2 cups

- ⅔ cup dried cramp bark (*Viburnum opulus*)
- ½ cup dried *Lobelia inflata*
- 3 cups rubbing alcohol
- 10 drops clary sage essential oil
- 10 drops Roman chamomile essential oil
- 5 drops geranium essential oil

1 Combine cramp bark, *Lobelia inflata*, and rubbing alcohol in a quart-sized Mason jar. Secure with a lid and label with the date and the ingredients. Shake the jar and place it on a sunny windowsill to infuse 4 weeks. Shake the jar vigorously a few times per week.

2 After the mixture is finished steeping, strain through a fine-mesh sieve lined with cheesecloth into a second quart-sized Mason jar or a spouted liquid measuring cup large enough to hold 1 quart of liquid. Add the essential oils to the strained alcohol and stir to combine.

3 To store, you can either return the alcohol to its original jar (after wiping out any residual herb pieces with a paper towel) or pour into smaller bottles fitted with spray tops for easy application. The finished liniment will maintain full potency for 1 year but will still be safe to use for up to 5 years.

4 Shake before using. To apply, either spritz the liniment directly on tight muscles or use a cotton ball to dab it on the skin. Either way, apply it liberally for best results.

Gua Sha: Coconut Oil "Scraping"

BENEFITS AND USES: *nearly instant relief of tight muscles*

AVOID: *if you have fragile skin, open sores, or a bleeding or clotting disorder, or if you are taking blood thinners*

YIELDS: 1 treatment

- 1 tablespoon coconut oil
- 1 smooth spoon, coin, or lid

1 Massage coconut oil into the area where you're experiencing muscle tension.

2 Using a quick, firm scraping motion, scrape the affected areas with a clean spoon, coin, or lid. Use just enough pressure for this to feel intense but not at all painful. Concentrate your strokes on the fleshy part of the muscles and never scrape over a bony prominence (this hurts!) or the front or sides of the neck.

3 After a few strokes, notice where you see redness or purple or red dots (petechiae) appear on the skin's surface. Areas that respond this way are the ones that benefit most from this technique. Continue to scrape, following the redness out to the sides as far as it will go, still making sure to avoid any bony spots.

4 After you've completed the scraping, your muscles will feel immediate relief. Keep the area warm and covered for 24 hours following treatment.

remedy notes

This technique works via counterirritation. The irritation caused by the scraping creates a small, controlled inflammation, which draws oxygenated blood to tissues that have been deprived of circulation. Be aware that redness and marks may remain visible on your skin for multiple days after the treatment. Note: This technique is safe for healthy adults. Do not apply it to children, elders, or people with chronic illness unless directed to do so by a healthcare provider.

Tea Tree Antifungal Spray

BENEFITS AND USES: *prevents and relieves mild fungal infections of the skin, including athlete's foot*

AVOID: *using on open cuts, on diabetic foot ulcers or wounds that are taking too long to heal, internally, or on the genital region*

YIELDS: 1 (2-ounce) bottle

▸ **¼ cup rubbing alcohol**

▸ **15 drops tea tree essential oil**

▸ **1 (2-ounce capacity) spray bottle**

1 Combine the rubbing alcohol and essential oil in the spray bottle. Shake well to combine. Store at cool room temperature and use within 2 months.

2 To use, spray the mixture over affected areas and allow to air dry. Repeat two to three times per day until the condition clears up. Keep the area as dry as possible between applications.

remedy notes

Tea tree essential oil boasts potent antifungal properties, but this formula's efficacy depends just as much on the rubbing alcohol used to dilute it. Unlike carrier oils, rubbing alcohol evaporates quickly and leaves the skin dry, depriving the fungus of the warm, moist environment it prefers.

✈ Pain-Relieving Cayenne Liniment ✈

BENEFITS AND USES: *relieves pain and stiffness that is eased by warmth and worsened by cold*

AVOID: *using internally or on open wounds, diabetic ulcers, or wounds that are taking too long to heal*

YIELDS: 50–75 applications

- 2 heaping tablespoons cayenne pepper
- ¼ cup (packed) fresh rosemary sprigs
- 6" knob or 2 ounces fresh ginger root, peeled and sliced
- 2 fresh habanero peppers (including the seeds), split in half lengthwise
- 2 cups rubbing alcohol
- 20 drops clary sage essential oil

1 Combine all ingredients except for the essential oil in a quart-sized Mason jar and cover with a lid. Label with the date and the ingredients. Shake well and place on a sunny windowsill to infuse 4 weeks. Shake vigorously a few times per week.

2 After the mixture is finished steeping, strain through a fine-mesh sieve lined with cheesecloth into another Mason jar or a spouted liquid measuring cup large enough to hold 2 cups of liquid. Add the essential oil to the strained alcohol and stir to combine. You can either return the liniment to the original jar after straining or pour into smaller bottles fitted with spray tops for ease of application.

3 Shake before each use. To apply, you can either spritz the liniment directly on painful areas or use a cotton ball to dab onto the skin.

St. John's Wort Oil for Chronic Pain

BENEFITS AND USES: *reduces nerve pain associated with shingles and Epstein-Barr*

AVOID: *N/A*

YIELDS: 1 application (for 5 square inches of skin)

▸ ½ teaspoon St. John's Wort–infused oil

Apply oil directly to areas where you're experiencing nerve pain or an outbreak of shingles and massage into skin until absorbed. Reapply as often as needed.

remedy notes

Best-quality St. John's Wort–infused oil is made with the fresh flowering plant at the height of midsummer. When it's made properly, the oil will have a deep ruby color. Don't purchase oil that wasn't made from fresh plants and doesn't have the characteristic color; it won't be effective.

Chapter 9

DETOXIFICATION AND DAMAGE CONTROL

Detoxification is a broad term for all of the ways your body eliminates waste products. From the visible parts of the process, like going to the bathroom, to the invisible reactions that take place in your liver and kidneys, detoxification is accomplished by a set of normal bodily functions. It doesn't require restrictive cleansing programs or strenuous regimens. If you reduce your chemical exposure when you can and supply your organs with the nutrients they need, the physical part of detox will take care of itself.

The safest approach to supporting detoxification is also most effective in the long run: eat simple meals made from whole plants without severely restricting yourself. You'll find recipes in this chapter for wholesome food and supportive remedies that supply your body with the nutrients you need for your liver, kidneys, large intestine, lungs, and skin to perform at their best. And for those times when you can't maintain an ideal diet, celebrate a little too hard, or just don't feel like yourself, you can turn to this chapter for simple ways to mitigate the damage.

☙ Ayurvedic Kitchari Cleanse ☙

BENEFITS AND USES: *gives your body a break after overindulging, while you're sick, or if you need to hit the "reset" button on your relationship with food*

AVOID: *if you have migraines that are triggered by turmeric; using as a cleanse if you have a history of disordered eating*

YIELDS: 8 servings

- 1 cup dried mung beans
- ½ cup brown rice
- ¼ teaspoon sea salt
- Water to fill
- 2 tablespoons unrefined sesame oil
- 2 teaspoons ground turmeric
- 1 tablespoon ground cumin
- 1 tablespoon ground coriander
- 2 cups baby spinach, tightly packed
- ½ cup cilantro leaves, chopped
- ½ small lemon, cut in half

1 Place mung beans, rice, and sea salt in a pot and add water until beans and rice are completely covered (with 1"–2" water above the level of the beans and rice). Bring to a boil, reduce to a simmer, and cook uncovered until rice and beans are soft. There will still be water in the pot.

2 Place oil and spices in a frying pan and warm over medium heat, stirring occasionally with a wooden spoon until the spices become fragrant, about 5 minutes.

Ayurvedic Kitchari Cleanse—continued

3 Use a slotted spoon to add the cooked rice and beans to the frying pan without adding too much of any remaining cooking water. Stir well to coat the mixture with the toasted spices. Add spinach and continue to cook over medium heat 5–6 more minutes until the spinach is wilted. Remove from heat and top with cilantro and a squeeze of fresh lemon juice.

4 To use as a cleanse, simply replace your regular meals and snacks with kitchari for 1–3 days. Make sure to eat enough kitchari to satisfy your hunger and drink plenty of fluids.

Kitchari is an Ayurvedic healing food that strikes the perfect balance between giving your system a "rest" and ensuring that you get all of your nutritional needs met so that you won't have to worry about rebound binge eating, low energy, or cravings.

Creamy Broccoli Soup

YIELDS: 6 servings

- 2 tablespoons extra-virgin olive oil
- 1 large white or yellow onion, peeled and chopped
- 1 large carrot, peeled and chopped
- 8 cloves garlic, peeled and chopped
- 6 cups water
- 1 pound broccoli, chopped
- 1 medium Yukon gold potato, scrubbed and cubed
- ¾ cup nutritional yeast
- 1 teaspoon dry mustard powder
- 4 large tongue depressor–shaped pieces astragalus root
- 1 cup roasted salted cashews, soaked overnight in water
- 3 tablespoons miso paste
- ½ teaspoon sea salt
- Juice of 1 lemon
- ⅛ teaspoon cayenne pepper
- About 2 tablespoons smoked paprika, divided

1 Warm olive oil in a large pot over medium heat for 2 minutes. Add onion and carrot. Cook until softened, stirring occasionally, about 5 minutes. Add the chopped garlic and cook another 2 minutes.

2 Add the water, broccoli, potato, yeast, mustard powder, and astragalus root. Increase heat to high and bring to a strong simmer and then reduce the heat to low and simmer gently for 15 minutes.

Creamy Broccoli Soup—continued

3 Turn off the heat. Remove astragalus pieces and discard. Remove 1 cup liquid from the pot and add to a high-speed blender along with cashews, miso, salt, lemon juice, and cayenne. Puree on low speed a few seconds and slowly increase to high speed. Puree on high speed until completely smooth, about 2–4 minutes depending on your blender.

4 If you prefer a chunky soup, add the cashew/miso cream to the pot, stir until combined, and then ladle into bowls to serve. Top each bowl with 1 teaspoon smoked paprika for extra color and flavor.

5 If you prefer a completely creamy soup, return the cashew/miso cream to the pot and stir. Then puree the soup in batches using the blender, or use an immersion blender to puree directly in the pot. Ladle into bowls and garnish each with about 1 teaspoon smoked paprika.

This soup combines the major "detox food groups" into one yummy formula. The alliums (onions and garlic), brassicas (broccoli), B vitamins (nutritional yeast), and citrus (lemon) each support a different aspect of detoxification. Mustard powder helps to activate beneficial compounds in broccoli, while cayenne stimulates digestion and circulation.

✈ Springtime Asparagus Soup ✈

YIELDS: 4 servings

- 1 tablespoon extra-virgin olive oil
- 1 large white or yellow onion, peeled and chopped
- 2 celery stalks, chopped
- ¼ teaspoon salt
- 2 small cloves garlic (or 1 large), peeled and chopped
- 1 small russet potato, peeled and chopped
- 3 cups chopped asparagus, 2" tips removed and set aside
- 5 cups water
- 1 tablespoon nutritional yeast
- ⅛ teaspoon cayenne pepper
- 1 tablespoon white miso paste
- 1 teaspoon freshly squeezed lemon juice

1 Warm oil in a soup pot over medium heat 2 minutes. Add onion, celery, and salt to the pot, stirring to coat the veggies with the oil.

2 Sweat vegetables over medium heat, stirring occasionally, until soft and translucent. If they start to brown, lower the heat. After 6 minutes, add garlic. Cook 1 more minute.

3 Add potato, asparagus, water, and nutritional yeast to the pot. Sprinkle cayenne pepper over the soup. Bring to a boil and then turn down to a simmer and partially cover. Simmer, partially covered, 20 minutes or until potato pieces are fork-tender and starting to fall apart.

4 Remove from heat and allow soup to cool slightly before adding miso paste and lemon juice. Working in batches if necessary, transfer soup to a blender and puree until smooth, or use an immersion blender.

✈ Golden Ginger Dressing ✈

BENEFITS AND USES: *supports liver detoxification, counteracts inflammation, and ensures optimal absorption of the nutrients contained in fresh greens*

AVOID: *if you're taking blood thinners*

YIELDS: about 1 cup

- ¼ cup apple cider vinegar
- ¼ cup extra-virgin olive oil
- ¼ cup toasted sesame oil
- 3 large cloves garlic, peeled
- 1½ tablespoons peeled and minced or grated fresh ginger root
- 2 teaspoons Turmeric Paste (see Chapter 8)
- 1 tablespoon miso paste
- 2 medjool dates, pitted
- Juice of 1 lime
- ¼ cup water
- ½ teaspoon salt
- ⅛ teaspoon cayenne pepper

Combine all ingredients in a blender and process on high speed until smooth, about 2–4 minutes. Dressing will keep in the fridge up to 1 week.

remedy notes

Serve this dressing on salad greens or steamed veggies for a nourishing side dish. For a quick, affordable, and healthy meal, use this dressing to make a warm grain, bean, and greens bowl. For each bowl, add ½ cup cooked brown rice, ½ cup cooked (or canned) beans, and 1–2 cups cooked or raw baby spinach. Top with Golden Ginger Dressing and garnish with hemp or sunflower seeds.

Kale Salad
with Instant Avocado Dressing

YIELDS: 2 servings

- ½ red onion, peeled and sliced into thin half moons
- Juice of 1 lime
- ½ teaspoon salt
- 1 large bunch kale, destemmed and chopped
- 1 ripe avocado, pitted and cut in half, divided
- 2 tablespoons liquid aminos (or use tamari or soy sauce)
- ½ cup hulled hemp seeds
- 2 tablespoons nutritional yeast

1 Place red onion in a small dish and cover with lime juice and salt. Toss to combine and set aside.

2 Place kale in a large bowl.

3 Cube ½ avocado and add to the bowl with the kale. Reserve the other avocado half to add at the end. Pour liquid aminos over kale and avocado.

4 Using clean hands, vigorously massage liquid aminos and avocado into kale. You want the kale to soften and wilt, so massage thoroughly about 5 full minutes. When you're done, the kale will be bright green, soft, and coated with the dressing.

5 Slice remaining avocado half into 1" cubes, add to the bowl, and toss to combine. To serve, divide salad between two serving bowls and top each with half the pickled red onions, hemp seeds, and nutritional yeast.

Garlic and Turmeric Spread

BENEFITS AND USES: *helps you get the detoxification-supporting, cancer-fighting, and anti-inflammatory benefits of turmeric and garlic into your regular diet*

AVOID: *if you're taking blood thinners or if you have FODMAP-sensitive IBS and/or a thick yellow coating on your tongue*

YIELDS: about ½ cup

- ½ cup roasted salted cashews, soaked overnight in water and drained
- 1 tablespoon miso paste
- 2 teaspoons Turmeric Paste (see Chapter 8)
- 2 teaspoons apple cider vinegar
- ½ tablespoon Italian seasoning
- 3 tablespoons Better Than Garlic Butter (see Chapter 8)
- 4 tablespoons water, divided

1 Add cashews, miso, Turmeric Paste, apple cider vinegar, Italian seasoning, Better Than Garlic Butter, and 3 tablespoons of the water to a blender. Blend 1 minute, starting on low speed and quickly increasing to high. Then stop and scrape down the sides of the blender. If mixture looks like it's too thick to blend easily, add remaining tablespoon of water.

2 Blend again (starting on low and increasing to high) about 60–90 seconds. Check the spread again, scraping down the sides of the blender if there are any bits of cashew that still haven't been incorporated. Repeat this process until the spread is smooth. Store finished spread in the fridge up to 10 days.

Turmeric, Cayenne, and Lemon Shot

BENEFITS AND USES: *clears the fog of a hangover, relieves pain, and supplies your liver with the nutrients it needs to detoxify your blood*

AVOID: *if you have gastroesophageal reflux disease (GERD) or are taking blood thinners*

YIELDS: 1 serving

- 1 clove garlic, peeled
- ½ teaspoon Turmeric Paste (see Chapter 8)
- Juice of 1 lemon
- ⅛ teaspoon cayenne pepper
- 1 tablespoon apple cider vinegar
- 1" knob fresh ginger root, peeled and sliced

1 Combine all ingredients in a high-speed blender. Blend on high 1–2 minutes, until smooth. If your blender is too large to effectively blend this small volume of ingredients, you can double the recipe or add ½ cup water to dilute.

2 Pour into a shot glass and drink immediately. It will be sour, strong, and spicy! Follow with plenty of water or the Citrus and Sea Salt Electrolyte Replenisher (see Chapter 8).

remedy notes

If you can tolerate more heat, feel free to increase the ginger and/or cayenne in this recipe. Both will help relieve pain and revive your energy. Ginger is especially helpful if you're suffering from a morning-after headache.

Activated Charcoal for Hangover Relief

BENEFITS AND USES: *reduces the intoxicating effects of alcohol and subsequent hangover symptoms*

AVOID: *if you're taking any form of prescription medication without consulting your doctor or pharmacist first*

YIELDS: 1 serving

▸ **1 (500-milligram) activated charcoal capsule per 100 pounds of body weight**

▸ **1 cup water**

Take capsule(s) with a full glass of water before drinking alcohol. If the charcoal is in your system when you start drinking, it may adsorb enough of the alcohol to prevent it from affecting you. As an alternative, you can take the capsule(s) after imbibing, but the effect won't be as strong.

remedy notes

This remedy is safe only for very occasional use; use no more than once per month. Activated charcoal can adsorb (bind to) a wide range of substances in the digestive tract and prevent your body from absorbing them—including nutrients and medications. Taking it regularly can cause serious nutrient deficiencies or encourage an unhealthy relationship with alcohol.

Ginger Juice Shot for Migraines

BENEFITS AND USES: *prevents migraines*

AVOID: *if you're taking blood thinners*

YIELDS: about 7 servings

- 2 large knobs fresh ginger root (about 8 ounces each), peeled and cut into 6 slices each
- 2 large apples, cored and cut into large slices

---

1 Add a slice of ginger root to a juicer, followed by a slice of apple. Continue alternating ginger and apple until you've juiced all ingredients. If your juicer can tolerate it, run the pulp through the juicer a second time to extract any remaining juice.

2 Pour the juice into an empty ice cube tray and freeze until solid. After the juice cubes are frozen, remove from the ice cube trays and store in a zip-top freezer bag so they'll stay as fresh as possible until you need them.

3 To use, remove 1–2 ice cubes from the freezer bag (enough to equal roughly 2 tablespoons of juice) and thaw in the microwave or on the stovetop until liquefied. Drink the shot. You can dilute slightly with ¼ cup water, if needed. Take this remedy as soon as possible after you feel the onset of a migraine aura.

remedy notes

Ginger juice can stop a migraine in its tracks if you take it right away, but it's less effective once you're experiencing a full-blown headache. Be sure to prepare this remedy before you need it so that it will be ready and waiting for you anytime you feel a headache coming on. Not only does ginger have anti-inflammatory and pain-relieving properties, but it's also a powerful circulatory stimulant. This remedy may work its magic by helping to normalize blood flow to the brain.

⋇ Antioxidant Smoothie ⋇

BENEFITS AND USES: *supplies your body with abundant micro-nutrients, antioxidants, and cancer-preventing phytonutrients and replenishes your iron*

AVOID: *N/A*

YIELDS: 2 servings

▸ Juice of 1 organic lemon, plus ¼ of lemon peel (yellow part only, avoid white pith)

▸ ½ cup fresh or frozen blueberries

▸ 1 cup fresh or frozen pitted cherries

▸ ⅔ cup frozen banana slices (equal to 1 medium banana)

▸ 2 cups baby spinach, packed

▸ 2 medjool dates, pitted

▸ ⅛ teaspoon cinnamon

▸ 1 cup water

Place all ingredients in a blender. Blend on high 2–4 minutes until smooth. Serve immediately.

Swap out the ingredients in this recipe to create endless variations. For example, try tropical fruits like mango and pineapple instead of the berries and pair them with a lime and some fresh ginger instead of the lemon and cinnamon. No matter what variations you try, always include the frozen banana slices. They're the secret to creating a creamy texture.

Cinnamon and Fenugreek Blood Sugar Shot

BENEFITS AND USES: *optimizes blood sugar response and increases insulin sensitivity*

AVOID: *if you have gastroesophageal reflux disease (GERD) or acid reflux that's triggered by vinegar*

YIELDS: 1 serving

> 1 teaspoon whole fenugreek seeds
> 1 teaspoon ground cinnamon
> 1 tablespoon apple cider vinegar
> 1 cup water

1 Grind fenugreek seeds with a mortar and pestle or coffee grinder.

2 Combine fenugreek, cinnamon, and apple cider vinegar in a shot glass.

3 Stir the shot vigorously and drink. If it takes more than one swallow for you to drink the whole shot, you might need to stir it before each sip. After taking the shot, drink a glass of water to clear the taste from your mouth. (If you prefer, you can dilute the shot in the glass of water instead. If you choose this method, drink the full glass within 10 minutes.)

4 For best results, use once per day and consume 15 minutes before your largest meal.

remedy notes

This shot is an efficient way to combine three natural ingredients proven to benefit blood sugar regulation. Since you need to take this remedy daily, it's convenient to partially prepare it in advance. For a week's worth of shots, grind 2½ tablespoons whole fenugreek seeds and combine with 2½ tablespoons ground cinnamon. Store the spice mixture in a labeled airtight container next to your apple cider vinegar. Add 2 teaspoons spice mixture per 1 tablespoon apple cider vinegar to prepare a single serving in seconds.

Dandelion Root Liver Cleanse

BENEFITS AND USES: *helps with cystic acne, PMS, mild depression with irritability, and constipation*

AVOID: *if you're taking any prescription medications (check with your doctor)*

YIELDS: 2 servings

> **3 heaping tablespoons dandelion root pieces**

> **4 cups water**

---

1. Add dandelion root and water to a small pot. Cover and bring to a rolling boil; then uncover and reduce heat to a simmer. Simmer 20 minutes. Strain and serve.

2. For best results, drink two servings of this decoction per day at least 6 days of the week. If you have hormonal acne, PMS, or other symptoms of an overburdened liver, do this for 3–4 weeks and track your symptoms. If this remedy doesn't make a difference after 1 month of consistent use, reach out to a clinical herbalist and/or medical professional.

remedy notes

If you want to enjoy the benefits of dandelion root but have trouble warming up to its bitter flavor, try making dandelion root chai. Add 1 small cinnamon stick, 2–3 slices fresh ginger, 2–3 cardamom pods, 1–2 whole cloves, and maybe even some fennel or star anise to this basic dandelion root decoction recipe. After simmering the decoction, add almond, hemp, or coconut milk to mellow the flavor even more, and sweeten with a teaspoon of maple syrup or honey, if desired.

⤜ Cinnamon Tea ⤛

YIELDS: 4 servings

- 1 cinnamon stick
- 1 tablespoon ground cinnamon
- 4 cups water
- 1 tablespoon blackstrap molasses

1 Add cinnamon stick, cinnamon, and water to a small pot and bring to a boil. Reduce heat to a gentle simmer and partially cover. Continue to simmer, partially covered, 15 minutes.

2 Remove cinnamon stick, stir in molasses, and serve. Store any leftover tea in a covered container in the refrigerator up to 48 hours. Drink 1–2 cups per day.

remedy notes

Most of the cinnamon on the market is *Cinnamomum cassia*, which contains a compound called coumarin that can cause liver damage in some people. This isn't a problem with normal culinary use, but if you're taking a medicinal dose of cinnamon over a long period of time, it's worth considering. To be on the safe side, avoid this remedy if you have any form of liver disease, or choose "sweet cinnamon" (*Cinnamomum verum*) from a bulk herb supplier to sidestep the coumarin issue altogether.

✈ Coconut Oil Roasted Sweet Potatoes ✈

BENEFITS AND USES: *prevents sugar cravings and helps the body let go of an addiction to refined sugars*

AVOID: *N/A*

YIELDS: 4 servings

- ▸ 2 tablespoons extra-virgin coconut oil, warmed until liquefied, plus more to grease pan
- ▸ 2 pounds sweet potatoes, cut into ½" wedges
- ▸ 2 teaspoons sea salt

1 Preheat oven to 400°F. Lightly coat a roasting pan or oven-safe dish with coconut oil.

2 Add sweet potato wedges to the prepared pan and toss with liquefied coconut oil. Roast 45 minutes, turning once at about the 25-minute mark. After turning, continue to roast for another 20–30 minutes, until potatoes are fork-tender and slightly crispy on the outside.

3 Remove from oven and sprinkle with sea salt. Serve warm and eat slowly to maximize your enjoyment.

remedy notes

Chinese medicine teaches that the "sweet" flavor is meant to be a foundational part of a healthy diet. Of course, this doesn't mean that refined sugar is healthful, but it can help to explain why cravings for sweet-tasting foods are so common and hard to quell. Instead of battling sugar cravings with willpower alone, try a sustainable approach that includes healthy, whole food sources of sweetness like this recipe. After about 2–3 weeks, your palate will start to adjust and you'll find it much easier to avoid refined sugars.

✦ Almond-Stuffed Medjool Dates ✦

BENEFITS AND USES: *offers your body a satisfying alternative to candy or dessert*

AVOID: *bingeing on this recipe to reduce the risk of bloating and blood sugar spikes*

YIELDS: 1 serving
- **8 raw almonds**
- **1 medjool date, split in half lengthwise and pitted**
- **⅛ teaspoon sea salt, divided**

1 Press 4 almonds into each date half.

2 Sprinkle each stuffed date half with half the sea salt.

3 Enjoy with a cup of tea!

remedy notes

These little treats are so satisfying because they combine the healthy fat of the almonds with the intense sweetness of the dates and a touch of salt for contrast. Much of the processed food people eat today was engineered to overstimulate the pleasure centers in the brain with precise combinations of salt, fat, and sugar. This recipe echoes that same tactic without any refined sugar or artificial ingredients. It's an ideal way to gently transition away from processed sweets.

Lavender and Peppermint Headache Balm

BENEFITS AND USES: *reduces the severity of a stress-related headache*

AVOID: *N/A*

YIELDS: 8 (1-ounce) tins

- ½ **cup jojoba oil**
- ½ **cup extra-virgin olive oil**
- **2 tablespoons shaved or pelleted beeswax**
- **40 drops lavender essential oil**
- **30 drops peppermint essential oil**
- **8 (1-ounce) tins to hold finished salve**

1 Set up a double boiler by filling a medium pot with a few inches of hot water and situating a heat-safe glass bowl atop the pot. Make sure that the glass is not touching the water and turn the burner on low. Add the jojoba and olive oils and beeswax to the glass bowl and gently warm until the wax is just melted.

2 Remove from heat. Open empty tins and set them up in a row on the counter with a paper towel underneath to catch any spills.

3 Add essential oils to the liquefied oil and wax mixture and stir. Immediately pour into the tins and allow the balm to cool to room temperature before covering. While waiting for the balm to cool, label the top of each tin.

4 Do your best to keep the finished balm away from extreme temperatures, but don't be afraid to keep a tin in your purse. It will maintain peak potency for about 1 year but will still be useable for up to 3 years.

5 To use, apply to your temples, forehead, base of your skull, neck, and/or wrists whenever you need relief from a tension headache or stress.

⇥ Cardamom and Ginger Masala Chai ⇤

BENEFITS AND USES: *helps you avoid the urge to binge eat*

AVOID: *if you're taking blood thinners*

YIELDS: 6 servings

- 3" knob or 1 ounce fresh ginger root, peeled and sliced
- 12 green cardamom pods
- 5 cups water
- 4 tea bags black tea (regular or decaf)
- About 1½ cups unsweetened soy milk, divided
- 6 drops liquid stevia, divided

1 Combine ginger, cardamom, and water in a small pot on the stovetop. Bring to a full boil and then turn down heat and gently simmer for 10–15 minutes, until water is fragrant and has a slightly golden hue.

2 Turn off heat and add black tea bags. Let tea steep according to package directions to ensure an optimal brew for the tea you've chosen. After steeping, remove tea bags from pot and squeeze out as much liquid as you can before discarding.

3 To make one serving of chai, place a small strainer over your teacup. Then ladle about ¾ cup spiced chai into your cup/strainer. Lift out strainer, then add soy milk and 1 drop liquid stevia. Store leftover chai in the fridge up to 4 days. Just reheat and follow these instructions whenever you need a sweet little pick-me-up.

remedy notes

The urge to binge or overeat is often triggered by emotional pain, stress, or anxiety. If sipping a cup or two of this chai doesn't help to quell the urge, try any of the remedies in Chapter 7 that focus on relieving anxiety. These remedies work even better when paired with good psychotherapy to help you develop effective ways of coping that don't cause the physical and emotional harm of chronic binge eating.

Chapter 10

WOMEN'S HEALTH

Human hormonal cycles exist in a dynamic relationship with natural cycles much bigger than our bodies. Shifts in your consciousness, energy level, desires, and physicality are normal manifestations of moving in harmony with these natural cycles, some of which play out over the course of a 24-hour period, while others take decades to unfold. Learning to embrace and enjoy the fact that our bodies are always changing is one of the secrets to enjoying optimal reproductive and hormonal health at every stage of life.

Of course, there are times when a change in how you feel signals that something is amiss. That's where this chapter comes in. You'll find remedies to relieve ailments such as yeast infections and urinary tract infections. You'll also learn how to ease common discomforts associated with menstruation and menopause. The Ginger Root Compress and Black Haw and Yarrow Tincture will help you calm menstrual cramps, and following the steps in the PMS Protocol will help make your whole menstrual cycle more comfortable. This chapter also includes ways to support fertility.

Tending to your hormonal and reproductive health requires that you care for yourself as a whole person. It isn't just about cobbling together a slew of remedies for various complaints. Since reproductive and hormonal health encompasses your relationship to your body and your sexuality, this chapter also includes recipes for aphrodisiacs, sensual massage oil, and even a sexual lubricant. A natural approach to supporting women's health is a big enough topic to be worthy of its own book. Consider this chapter an introduction to the possibilities.

Red Raspberry Uterine Tonic

YIELDS: 3 servings

> 1 heaping cup dried red raspberry leaf

> 4 cups hot water

1 Add red raspberry leaf to a quart-sized Mason jar. Cover with hot water and stir until all of the herb is saturated. Then let the infusion steep on the counter at least 4 hours or overnight.

2 Strain through cheesecloth, a nut milk bag, or a fine-mesh sieve into a second Mason jar or pitcher. Make sure to squeeze the extra liquid out of the herbs!

3 Drink 1–2 cups per day for gentle, nourishing support of uterine health. Store any leftover infusion in the fridge up to 48 hours.

remedy notes

Red raspberry leaf has proven effects on the uterine muscle, including helping to relax chronic spasms and making uterine contractions more effective. This makes it a valuable remedy both for women who experience menstrual cramps and to help prepare the uterus for giving birth. This preparation is widely considered to be safe and beneficial during pregnancy, but consult with your doctor or midwife if you have any concerns. Because of its drying, astringent properties, red raspberry leaf may reduce your milk supply if you use it in large amounts while breastfeeding.

Restorative Gingerbread Latte

BENEFITS AND USES: *rebuilds energy and warmth when you feel depleted by blood loss associated with menstruation or childbirth*

AVOID: *N/A*

YIELDS: 1 serving

- ¼ cup hulled raw sunflower seeds
- 1 cup water
- 1 heaping tablespoon blackstrap molasses
- ¼ teaspoon dried ginger or 1 teaspoon grated fresh ginger root
- ¼ teaspoon ground cinnamon

---

1 Add sunflower seeds and water to a high-speed blender. Blend on high until completely smooth, about 60–90 seconds, depending on your equipment. Strain through a nut milk bag or fine-mesh sieve lined with cheesecloth into a bowl or liquid measuring cup. Rinse out the blender to remove any remaining solids and return the strained sunflower seed milk to the blender.

2 Add molasses, ginger, and cinnamon to the blender and process on medium until smooth and combined.

3 Serve hot or cold, according to your preference.

remedy notes

Many practitioners encourage women to consume red meat and organ meats to prevent or reverse anemia, but you can get enough iron to replenish yourself from plant-based sources if you prefer. Drink 3–4 quarts Stinging Nettle Infusion for Strong Hair, Nails, and Teeth (see Chapter 4) per week in combination with daily use of this recipe and enjoy iron-rich foods like lentils, cooked spinach, and pumpkin seeds.

Cranberry, Marshmallow, and Echinacea Cooler

YIELDS: 4 servings

FOR THE COOLER:

- 1 batch Soothing Marshmallow Root Infusion (see Chapter 6)
- ½ cup unsweetened 100 percent pure cranberry juice, divided
- 1 tablespoon echinacea tincture

FOR THE REST OF THE PROTOCOL:

- Additional ½ cup cranberry juice, divided
- 4 cups water, divided
- Additional 1½ teaspoons echinacea tincture, divided

1 As soon as you feel the first symptoms of a potential UTI, combine ½ teaspoon echinacea tincture, ⅛ cup 100 percent cranberry juice, and 1 cup water in a large glass. Drink the whole glass within 5 minutes, if possible.

2 While preparing the Soothing Marshmallow Root Infusion (about 4 hours), drink 1 (8-ounce) glass of water with ⅛ cup cranberry juice and 1 dropperful (¼ teaspoon) echinacea tincture added per hour.

3 Once the Soothing Marshmallow Root Infusion is ready, combine it with 1 tablespoon echinacea tincture and ½ cup cranberry juice in a large pitcher and stir.

4 Drink 1 (8-ounce) glass of the cooler every hour or two until symptoms improve. Then reduce frequency to 3–4 glasses per day until you've been completely symptom free for 3 days. After 3 days with no symptoms, you can discontinue the formula.

Cranberry, Marshmallow, and Echinacea Cooler—continued

5 On the first day you notice UTI symptoms, make sure that you not only consume an entire batch of this remedy but that you also start a second batch of Soothing Marshmallow Root Infusion before going to bed so it will be ready in the morning.

remedy notes

This protocol has a high rate of efficacy if you start it early enough and follow the instructions. If you delay your first dose, or if you don't drink enough of the remedies, it may not be enough to prevent the infection from worsening. If you're running a fever or experiencing back pain, flank pain, or blood in your urine (including blood on the toilet paper), your urinary tract infection might have progressed to a much more serious kidney infection. Seek medical care so that you won't risk permanent damage to your kidneys.

Essential Oil Bath Blend for UTI Relief

BENEFITS AND USES: *temporarily relieves pain and the feeling of urgency associated with a urinary tract infection*

AVOID: *if you're running a fever or experiencing back pain, flank pain, or blood in your urine (or on the toilet paper). Seek medical care instead.*

YIELDS: 1 bath

- 7 drops Roman chamomile essential oil
- 5 drops geranium essential oil
- 5 drops lavender essential oil
- 3 drops tea tree essential oil

1 Draw a hot bath, making sure that the temperature isn't too hot to sit in comfortably.

2 Add essential oils to the bath. Using your hands, vigorously "stir" the oils into the bathwater for 30–60 seconds before entering the bath.

3 Soak for 20–30 minutes or until the water becomes lukewarm. Repeat as often as desired.

remedy notes

This bath blend relies on the antispasmodic action of Roman chamomile to relieve the involuntary muscle spasms that cause the urge to urinate even when your bladder is empty. The antimicrobial effects of tea tree essential oil combined with the calming, balancing properties of geranium and lavender round out the formula. On its own, this bath won't treat your UTI, but it's a great source of temporary relief while you're waiting for either the Cranberry, Marshmallow, and Echinacea Cooler or physician-prescribed antibiotics to kick in.

Garlic Pessary
for Vaginal Yeast Infections

YIELDS: 1 pessary
- 1 clove garlic, gently peeled
- 1 (6") piece sterile medical gauze

1 Place garlic in the center of the strip of gauze and wrap the gauze around the garlic two or three times. Hold the garlic clove, twist the "tail" of gauze, and tie it into a tight knot just below the garlic. Double-check the knot to ensure that the garlic is secure and that you've tied the knot tightly enough to leave a "tail" of gauze at one end to help make it easier to remove the pessary after use.

2 Insert the gauze-wrapped garlic into your vagina in the evening, before bed. Do not have penetrative intercourse or insert anything else into the vagina while the pessary is in place. Remove in the morning and repeat the following night with a new pessary if symptoms are not completely gone. (It's normal to taste garlic in your mouth during and for a few hours after using this remedy.)

remedy notes

All natural remedies for yeast infections are not created equal. Stick with the garlic and avoid using essential oils or coconut oil internally. For best results, use the pessary in combination with a good probiotic supplement that includes both *Lactobacillus rhamnosus* and *Lactobacillus reuteri* while removing as much refined sugar from your diet as possible.

Mullein and Sage Tea

BENEFITS AND USES: *helps to relieve a yeast infection*

AVOID: *if you are taking blood thinners or pharmaceutical diuretics*

YIELDS: 2 servings

- 1 heaping tablespoon dried mullein leaf
- 1 teaspoon dried sage leaf
- 2 cups hot water

---

1 Measure the herbs into a tea ball, paper tea filter, or teapot fitted with a strainer. If using a tea ball or filter, add to your favorite mug. Add hot water, cover, and steep 20 minutes before serving.

2 For best results, drink 3–4 cups per day while symptoms persist and use in combination with the Garlic Pessary for Vaginal Yeast Infections (see recipe in this chapter).

remedy notes

Herbs are versatile. Mullein is soothing to all of the epithelial tissue in the body, which is why it shows up in formulas to help the lungs, the digestive tract, and the urogenital tract. Sage's antimicrobial properties are just as effective against vaginal infections as they are against upper respiratory infections.

⤛ Red Clover Infusion ⤜

BENEFITS AND USES: *cools hot flashes and mood swings associated with perimenopause and menopause*

AVOID: *if you have a personal or family history of estrogen-dependent cancer or are taking blood thinners*

YIELDS: 3 servings
- **1 heaping cup dried red clover leaf**
- **4 cups hot water**

1   Add red clover leaf to a quart-sized Mason jar. Pour hot water over the herbs and stir until all of the plant material is saturated.

2   Let the infusion steep on the counter at least 4 hours or overnight.

3   Strain through cheesecloth, a nut milk bag, or a fine-mesh strainer into a second Mason jar or a pitcher. Make sure to squeeze all of the liquid out of the herbs! Store any leftover infusion in the fridge and consume within 48 hours.

4   Serve hot or chilled, according to your preference. Drink 1–2 cups per day for gentle, nourishing support during menopause.

remedy notes

Phytoestrogen means "plant estrogen," but it's a little bit of a misnomer. Phytoestrogens aren't the same as human hormones; they just have a similar chemical structure and shape. This similar shape allows them to occupy some of the receptor sites that are crying out for estrogen during menopause. Think of them as a way to "stretch" your own estrogen supply. With regular consumption of this infusion and other sources of phytoestrogens, like flaxseed, tofu, tempeh, edamame, and sesame seeds, you may notice a reduction in hot flashes within 1 month.

Black Haw and Yarrow Tincture

YIELDS: about 2 cups

- ¼ cup dried black haw bark (*Viburnum prunifolium*)
- ¼ cup dried yarrow
- 2" knob fresh ginger root, peeled and minced
- ⅛ cup dried dandelion root
- 1 tablespoon dried licorice root
- ¼ cup boiling water
- 3 cups 100-proof vodka

1 Add the herbs to a quart-sized Mason jar. Pour water over herbs. Stir and let stand 15 minutes.

2 Pour vodka over damp herb mixture. Cover with a lid and clearly label the jar. Give the jar a good shake and set aside 24 hours.

3 Check on your tincture the next day. The herbs should be swelling as they absorb the vodka, but there should always be at least 3" vodka above the level of the herbs. If the herbs are creeping too close to the top of the jar, add another ½ cup vodka.

4 Let the tincture steep at least 3 weeks and up to 6 weeks. Shake the jar a few times per week, if possible, and keep an eye on the level of the liquid. Top off the jar with a little bit more vodka as needed.

Black Haw and Yarrow Tincture—continued

5 When the formula is finished infusing, strain it through a fine-mesh sieve into another quart-sized jar or large liquid measuring cup. Bottle and label the tincture. Store at cool room temperature away from sunlight. Its potency will slowly degrade after 1 year, but it will still be safe to use for up to 5 years.

6 To use, take ½ teaspoon in a small amount of water (at least ⅛ cup) as often as needed to relieve menstrual cramps.

Traditional Chinese Medicine compares herbs in a formula with roles people play in society. To update the metaphor, we can compare the herbs to people at a meeting. Black haw and yarrow are like co-presidents; they're in charge of addressing the main complaint. Dandelion is like an executive assistant supporting the co-presidents. Ginger is like the facilitator, encouraging good circulation to guide the formula where it's needed. Licorice is sweet and works like tea and cookies at a board meeting. A tiny amount harmonizes the formula and helps the other herbs to get along.

Ginger Root Compress

BENEFITS AND USES: *relieves menstrual cramps, especially when accompanied by dark red or brown blood and clots*

AVOID: *during pregnancy*

YIELDS: 1 treatment

- 6" knob or 2 ounces fresh ginger root, peeled and finely chopped
- 2 cups water
- 2 washcloths or hand towels
- Heating pad or hot water bottle

1 Add ginger and water to a small pot and bring to a boil; then reduce heat to a simmer and partially cover. Simmer, partially covered, 20 minutes.

2 Let the liquid cool a little. You want it to be very warm but not hot enough to burn your skin. Strain the liquid into a heat-safe container and immediately return it to the pot.

3 Soak one washcloth or hand towel in the ginger liquid and wring it out so that it's wet but not dripping. Apply the compress to the affected area and place the second (dry) washcloth or hand towel on top. Cover with a hot water bottle or heating pad.

4 Keep the compress on 20 minutes. If your symptoms have subsided after one round of the treatment, store the remaining liquid in the fridge up to 3 days just in case you need another treatment later in your cycle. If you still have cramps, you can warm up the ginger decoction again and repeat step 3 as many times as you desire.

 remedy notes

If your cramps are severe, use this treatment in combination with the Black Haw and Yarrow Tincture (see recipe in this chapter). You can also add ¼ cup black haw bark (*Viburnum prunifolium*) or cramp bark (*Viburnum opulus*) and 1 tablespoon cayenne pepper to this formula (along with an extra ¼ cup water) for an even stronger pain-relieving effect.

✦ Dandelion Leaf Tea ✦

BENEFITS AND USES: *encourages urination to relieve water retention*

AVOID: *if you are using blood thinners, lithium, or pharmaceutical diuretics*

YIELDS: 1 serving

- ⟩ **2 tablespoons dried dandelion leaf**
- ⟩ **2 cups hot water**

---

1 Add dandelion leaf to a quart-sized Mason jar. Cover with hot water and stir until all of the herb is saturated.

2 Steep 20 minutes and then strain through a fine-mesh sieve into a large mug or a second Mason jar and drink. You should notice an increase in urinary volume and frequency within 90 minutes.

3 If you're not back to normal the next day, take another dose of this remedy. Make sure to drink lots of water and eat a low-sodium diet too. If water retention persists, consult your healthcare provider.

remedy notes

Dandelion leaf and root offer different benefits, though both parts of the plant are bitter and cooling. The leaf is a potassium-sparing diuretic that's chock-full of nutrients while the root supports healthy liver function. Dandelion flowers offer benefits, too, and can be eaten as a food or infused into olive, sesame, or jojoba oil to make a wonderful massage oil for sore muscles.

Fresh Dandelion Leaf Tea
for Water Retention

BENEFITS AND USES: *relieves bloating and puffiness from water retention*

AVOID: *if you are taking diuretics, blood thinners, or blood pressure medication*

YIELDS: 1 serving

- ½ cup fresh dandelion leaves, washed and tightly packed
- 2½ cups water

1 Add dandelion leaves and water to a small pot. Bring to a boil and then reduce heat to a gentle simmer and cook 15 minutes or until the leaves are wilted and the water has a greenish tinge. Remove from heat.

2 Place a fine-mesh sieve over a teacup or mug and ladle the liquid into the mug using the sieve to catch any stray leaves. You can eat the spent leaves or discard them, according to your preference.

3 Drink the full recipe for best results. You should notice an increase in urinary volume and frequency within 90 minutes. If you're not back to normal the next day, take another dose of this remedy. Make sure to drink lots of water and eat a low-sodium diet too. If water retention persists, consult your healthcare provider.

remedy notes

Knowing how to make dandelion leaf tea with both fresh and dried leaves makes it possible to get quick relief from water retention even when you don't have access to a well-stocked herb cupboard or a natural food store. Once you experience their many medicinal properties, you might notice that you're less irritated by their ubiquity than when you thought of dandelions as little more than pesky weeds. You'll know you've really become an herb enthusiast when you catch yourself smiling at the heroic little dandelions pushing their way up through cracks in the sidewalk.

⊱ PMS Protocol ⊰

BENEFITS AND USES: *balances your energy and hormones so you can thrive during all phases of your menstrual cycle*

AVOID: *N/A*

YIELDS: improved hormonal balance

- **Simple Sunrise Medicine, daily (see Chapter 7)**
- **1 cup Dandelion Root Liver Cleanse, daily (see Chapter 9)**
- **20–30 minutes daily exercise**
- **1 batch Skullcap and Kuzu Root Tension Reliever (see Chapter 7)**
- **1–2 Dead Sea Salt Bath for Stress Relief (see Chapter 7)**
- **Muscle-Loving Omega-3 Brownie Bites (see Chapter 8)**
- **Avocado Cacao Truffles (see recipe in this chapter)**

---

1 How you care for yourself during the time when you're not menstruating has a major effect on your period. Spending time with the sun helps to reset your hormones, including your thyroid hormones and your reproductive hormones. Drinking dandelion root tea helps your liver to remove excess hormones from your bloodstream and will make your premenstrual week much, much easier. Regular exercise boosts your mood, circulates your body's vital energy, and improves pelvic circulation to reduce cramping.

2 During PMS, have resources on hand to make your life easier and more comfortable. The Skullcap and Kuzu Root Tension Reliever might not taste great, but it works like magic on PMS-induced feelings of anger, frustration, and muscle tension. Dead Sea Salt Bath for Stress Relief is a healthy way to unwind and take time for yourself. Chocolate cravings often signal that your body needs magnesium and "feel-good" neurochemicals. Ignoring your cravings can lead to binges, especially when your willpower is weakened by physical or emotional discomfort. Treat yourself with healthy options like the Muscle-Loving Omega-3 Brownie Bites and Avocado Cacao Truffles.

⤙ Aphrodisiac Oxymel ⤚

BENEFITS AND USES: *supports a healthy libido during times of stress*

AVOID: *if you have a history of schizophrenia, manic episodes, or a bleeding or clotting disorder, or if you're taking digoxin, antipsychotic medications, lithium, or blood thinners*

YIELDS: about ½ cup

- **2 tablespoons dried damiana leaf**
- **2 tablespoons dried eleuthero (*Eleutherococcus senticosus*) root**
- **½ tablespoon freshly grated nutmeg**
- **1 tablespoon cardamom pods or 1 teaspoon ground cardamom**
- **¼ cup plus 2 tablespoons water**
- **½ cup apple cider vinegar**
- **¼ cup plus 1 tablespoon raw honey**

1 Add damiana, eleuthero, nutmeg, cardamom, and water to a small pot. Warm over medium-low heat, stirring constantly, about 5 minutes or until herbs are fragrant and most of the water appears to be absorbed.

2 Add apple cider vinegar to herbs. Bring up to a very low simmer, give herbs a stir, and partially cover. Set a kitchen timer for 10 minutes and warm the mixture over low heat until the timer goes off. Keep the heat low enough so that mixture is barely bubbling.

3 When the timer goes off, turn off heat and cover the pot. Let sit another 10 minutes.

4 Strain the infused vinegar through a fine-mesh sieve into a liquid measuring cup. Once you squeeze out as much liquid as possible from the spent herbs, you should have approximately ¼ cup infused vinegar. Add an equal volume of raw honey to your infused vinegar and stir to combine. Bottle the finished oxymel and make sure to label it clearly.

Aphrodisiac Oxymel—continued

5 Take ½ tablespoon per day to support your libido during times of stress. If you need a little help getting in the mood, take an extra ½ tablespoon about 30 minutes before beginning sexual activity.

remedy notes

This formula is a restorative aphrodisiac. It might not have an immediate effect on your desire. Instead, it works over time to replenish the resources drained by libido killers like stress and fatigue. Eleuthero is an adaptogen that helps the body to recover from stress and build resilience. In scientific studies, damiana has been shown to increase sexual appetite and decrease the length of the refractory period (a period after intense stimulation when the body is not responsive to additional stimulation). Ultimately, aphrodisiacs are personal. Anything that helps you relax, open your heart, and experience sensory delight in the present moment has the potential to be an aphrodisiac.

Avocado Cacao Truffles

BENEFITS AND USES: *helps when served at the end of a romantic meal*

AVOID: *N/A*

YIELDS: about 12 truffles

- **5 medjool dates, pitted**
- **½ cup hot water**
- **Flesh of 1 medium avocado**
- **½ teaspoon ground cinnamon, divided**
- **½ teaspoon ground cardamom, divided**
- **5 tablespoons cacao powder, plus 1 tablespoon for coating**
- **1½ tablespoons melted coconut oil**
- **¼ teaspoon sea salt**
- **⅛ teaspoon large-flake sea salt**

1 Cover the dates with hot water and let stand 5 minutes.

2 Remove dates from water, reserving soaking water. Place dates in the bowl of a food processor with 2 tablespoons soaking water. Process about 3–4 minutes, until dates form a smooth paste. You can add up to 2 additional tablespoons date-soaking water and/or stop to scrape down the work bowl, if needed.

3 Add avocado, ¼ teaspoon of the cinnamon, ¼ teaspoon of the cardamom, 5 tablespoons cacao powder, melted coconut oil, and ¼ teaspoon sea salt to the food processor. Process until smooth. Chill in the fridge about 30 minutes or until the batter is firm enough to form into truffles.

4 Place remaining 1 tablespoon cacao powder in a shallow tray or dish. Add remaining ¼ teaspoon of cinnamon and ¼ teaspoon of cardamom. Stir to combine.

Avocado Cacao Truffles—continued

5 Form truffles by scooping out one rounded tablespoon of truffle batter at a time and forming into a ball. Drop each into the shallow bowl with the cacao powder and spices.

6 Roll each truffle in the powder until fully dusted. Sprinkle a pinch of large-flake sea salt over each truffle. Chill at least 30 minutes before serving. Store any leftovers in a parchment-lined tin or container in the fridge and consume within 48 hours.

remedy notes

Chocolate may be one of the world's most famous aphrodisiacs, but avocados have their own reputation as libido enhancers. Nutritionists consider the high levels of vitamin E in avocados to be beneficial for fertility, and a growing body of research shows that the fruit benefits cardiovascular health. What does heart health have to do with sex? For one thing, arterial plaques and atherosclerosis can impede pelvic circulation, reducing sexual pleasure and even causing erectile dysfunction in men. These truffles won't contribute to such problems, and they may even help to nudge things in the right direction.

⚘ Sensual Ginger and Coconut ⚘ Massage Oil

YIELDS: 1¼ cups

> **6" knob peeled and minced fresh ginger root**
> **1 cup extra-virgin coconut oil**
> **¼ cup jojoba oil**
> **20 drops nutmeg essential oil**

1 Combine ginger, coconut oil, and jojoba oil in a double boiler. Warm in the double boiler over simmering water for 2 hours. (Check the water level after 1 hour and add more if it's getting low.)

2 Strain infused oil through a fine-mesh sieve lined with cheesecloth. Discard spent ginger root. Add nutmeg essential oil.

3 Pour into a wide-mouthed jar (the wide mouth is important since this oil will be semi-solid at temperatures below 75°F and you won't be able to pour it to dispense). Label the jar and store at room temperature up to 1 year.

4 To use, massage into skin with relaxed hands using long, flowing strokes.

remedy notes

Sexual pleasure depends on your ability to notice and enjoy sensation. This massage oil encourages your body to release muscular tension that can block pleasurable sensation from touch, while the complex, yummy fragrance entrances your emotions through your sense of smell. If you use this oil regularly before sexual activity, your unconscious mind will build an association between this scent and the anticipation of pleasure. As that association becomes stronger, so will the aphrodisiac effects.

Aloe and Rose Water Lubricant

YIELDS: about 4 applications
- ¼ cup fresh aloe vera gel (see Aloe Vera recipe in Chapter 3)
- ⅛ cup rose water

1 Place aloe vera gel and rose water in a blender or food processor. Blend on high until completely smooth, about 1–3 minutes, depending on your equipment.

2 Store in the refrigerator in a covered container up to 1 week, or freeze in an ice cube tray so that you can defrost individual "servings" as needed.

3 To use as a personal lubricant, dispense 1–2 tablespoons of the gel into a clean dish and apply as needed. If using after refrigeration or freezing, be sure to let the gel return to room temperature before applying.

remedy notes

This is a safe alternative to the most popular natural lubricant: coconut oil. While coconut oil works beautifully as a personal lubricant for many people, it has two major downsides. First, coconut oil is incompatible with latex condoms. Second, it can increase the risk of vaginal yeast infections and bacterial vaginosis in some women. Aloe vera gel is water based, which means it resembles your body's natural lubrication more than an oil-based lubricant. It's also safe to use with latex condoms.

First Steps for Fertility

BENEFITS AND USES: *helps you approach your desire to conceive with self-compassion, openness, and ease*

AVOID: *if you and your partner have been trying to conceive for more than 1 year, if you have reproductive health issues, or if you are in your 40s or older. Instead, talk to your doctor.*

YIELDS: 1 week of fertility support

- Simple Sunrise Medicine, daily (see Chapter 7)
- Cycle tracking, daily (see step 2)
- 1 batch Stinging Nettle Infusion for Strong Hair, Nails, and Teeth (see Chapter 4)
- 3 batches Red Raspberry Uterine Tonic (see recipe in this chapter)
- Powerful Passionflower and Skullcap Tea, as needed for stress (see Chapter 7)

1 Practicing the Simple Sunrise Medicine exercise will help to balance your hormones by regulating your pineal and pituitary glands. It's effective, side effect–free, and 100 percent safe.

2 Use a fertility-tracking app every day to record your basal body temperature, cervical fluid, cervical position, and days of menstruation so that you can time intercourse to coincide with your fertile time each month.

3 Abundant nourishment is vital for preconception and fertility. Eat a diet that includes generous servings of vegetables, healthy fats, fruit, whole grains, and legumes. Include nourishing infusions to pack in even more nutrients (Stinging Nettle Infusion for Strong Hair, Nails, and Teeth) and to support uterine health (Red Raspberry Uterine Tonic). Drink 2 cups of infusion per day, aiming to consume three whole batches of Red Raspberry Uterine Tonic and 1 batch of Stinging Nettle Infusion for Strong Hair, Nails, and Teeth per week.

First Steps for Fertility—continued

4 Address your stress. Like all mammals, humans have built-in mechanisms that interfere with conception when the mother's body is under significant stress. Drink a cup of Powerful Passionflower and Skullcap Tea whenever you're feeling anxious or overwhelmed, and make use of exercise, journaling, and social support to manage the stress of wondering whether or not you will be able to conceive.

remedy notes

The rule of thumb I follow in my practice is that interventions that focus on women's reproductive hormones can take three full menstrual cycles to show their full effect. I'd encourage you to try these DIY fertility interventions for 3 months before jumping to any conclusions. After 3 months, you might decide that you're ready to seek additional help from an herbalist specializing in women's health or from a medical doctor (or both!).

Poke Root and Geranium Breast Oil

BENEFITS AND USES: *relieves congestion, swelling, and soreness associated with PMS*

AVOID: *if pregnant or breastfeeding*

YIELDS: about 1 cup

- ½ **cup extra-virgin olive oil**
- ½ **cup jojoba oil**
- ½ **cup chopped fresh poke root or ¼ cup dried**
- **40 drops geranium essential oil**

1 Place olive oil, jojoba oil, and poke root in a double boiler. Warm over low heat 2 hours, checking every 30 minutes to replenish water and ensure that oil doesn't get too hot. (If bubbles start to form in the oil, turn off heat and let cool 30 minutes before reapplying heat.) After 2 hours of infusing, let stand off heat until cool.

2 Strain through a fine-mesh sieve lined with cheesecloth into a small bowl or liquid measuring cup. Make sure to give the cheesecloth a good squeeze with your hands to extract as much of the medicated oil as possible. Dispose of the spent poke root so that pets and children won't get into it; it could make them sick if they ingest it.

3 Add geranium essential oil to the bottle you'll use to store the oil. (A pint-sized Mason jar would work well.) Pour the infused oil into the bottle using a funnel if needed and secure with a lid. Clearly label the bottle "Do not eat!" or "Not for internal use." Store at room temperature out of reach of children and use within 1 year.

4 To use the oil, apply liberally to the breasts and surrounding tissue. Massage each breast using upward circular motions, stroking toward the armpit, where the lymph nodes are located. Spend extra time on any areas that feel sore or congested.

Fenugreek Hilbe for Lactation Support

BENEFITS AND USES: *increases milk supply while breastfeeding*

AVOID: *eating too much of this remedy; consult your doctor before use if you're taking metformin or use insulin*

YIELDS: about 1 cup

- ⅛ cup whole fenugreek seeds
- Water, for soaking
- 2 cloves garlic, peeled
- Juice of 1 lemon
- ½ bunch (heaping ½ cup packed) chopped fresh cilantro leaves and stems
- ½ teaspoon salt
- ½ teaspoon ground cumin
- 1 tablespoon water

1 In a large bowl, soak fenugreek seeds in water 48 hours, changing the water once per day to reduce bitterness. After soaking fenugreek, rinse and drain it.

2 Add garlic cloves to the bowl of a food processor and process 30 seconds or until chopped. Add soaked fenugreek, lemon juice, cilantro, salt, and cumin to the food processor. Process 1 minute and then stop and scrape down the sides of the work bowl. Add 1 tablespoon water and process another 2–3 minutes, until mixture is completely smooth.

3 Serve as a dip for whole wheat pita bread, over warm chickpeas, or stirred into plain hummus. Store in a covered container in the fridge up to 1 week.

Cabbage Leaf Poultice

BENEFITS AND USES: *reduces breast engorgement and oversupply during lactation; prevents and treats mastitis*

AVOID: *using this treatment too frequently if you need to maintain a healthy supply of breastmilk*

YIELDS: 1 treatment

> 1 green cabbage leaf, chilled

1 Using a rolling pin, bruise cabbage leaf until slightly softened.

2 Place softened cabbage leaf against affected breast. If you want to use the treatment underneath your bra, cover cabbage leaf with a piece of clean fabric before putting inside your bra. Make sure that your bra isn't too tight, as this can contribute to mastitis.

3 Leave cabbage leaf on 20 minutes. Repeat treatment up to three times per day to help control engorgement.

remedy notes

If you are actively breastfeeding, start slowly with this remedy until you know how it will affect your milk supply. Use one treatment per breast per day to start, and increase slowly. If you are lactating but not breastfeeding and want to encourage your body to stop producing milk, use this treatment liberally and drink sage leaf tea.

NEXT STEPS AND RESOURCES

I hope that the recipes in this book have whet your appetite to learn more about natural medicine. An introductory book can carry you only a short way down the path, but I hope that what you can see on the horizon from here will entice you to keep going. In this section, I'm going to encourage you to keep learning and experimenting with herbal remedies and point the way toward some resources that can help you to deepen your knowledge.

You Have Permission to Experiment

When you first begin making your own herbal remedies, it's best to follow the directions exactly as written. Once you're comfortable with the process of making teas, tinctures, syrups, oxymels, and other preparations in this book, you might start to feel the urge to adapt the recipes a little bit. Maybe you want to add some ginger to a recipe that doesn't call for it, or maybe you're out of cinnamon and you want to see how the Elderberry Spice Syrup (see Chapter 5) would taste without any other spices besides the elderberries themselves. Go for it! Most of the recipes in this book can serve as templates for your experimentation and elaboration. Here are some guidelines to keep in mind when you're adapting recipes and making substitutions:

- Keep the ratios of liquid to solid ingredients intact. This same principle holds true for the ratios of liquid oils to coconut oil, wax, and solid butters in skincare preparations.
- When substituting herbs and spices, keep in mind not only the health-promoting function of the ingredient in the remedy but also the flavor and "temperature." For example, dandelion leaf is cold and bitter. Garlic is hot and pungent. Check the Remedy Notes or refer to a reliable materia medica (a reference book detailing the properties of medicinal herbs and their applications) for help identifying good substitutions.
- Change one ingredient at a time, whenever possible. If you change too many things at once, it will complicate your learning process.
- Keep notes on the changes that work—and the ones that don't. Your notes will help you recreate your best discoveries and avoid making the same mistake twice.

When you feel confident enough to adjust a remedy to suit the specific needs of the person you're making it for, you can experience a whole new level of efficacy and enjoyment. With a little bit more study and a splash of creativity, you can create a whole suite of custom remedies designed just for you and your beloveds.

When to See a Professional Herbalist

Throughout this book I've made suggestions about the kinds of situations that can be safely addressed by home remedies and distinguished them from those that require medical attention. There's a third category that I haven't covered: when to see a professional herbalist. The right herbalist can provide precise herbal support for conditions that are too complex or confusing for a DIY approach. An herbalist can often point you toward effective options when your doctor has run tests and been unable to find anything. And herbalists are the perfect people to consult if you don't have an illness or diagnosis but you know that you could feel healthier, more vibrant, and more like yourself.

How to Find an Herbalist

Unlike acupuncturists, dentists, and physicians, herbalists are not yet subject to governmental licensing requirements in the United States. That means there are no legal hoops for people to jump through before they're allowed to call themselves herbalists. For better or worse, the government has nothing to say on the matter of whether an herbalist is qualified to practice her art. While it's always a good idea to do your homework about any healthcare provider before trusting her with your health, the fact that herbalism remains an unlicensed profession means that it's up to you to decide whether or not any given practitioner has the necessary training and experience to do a good job. Here are some good questions to ask as you evaluate whether any particular herbalist is a good match for your needs.

- What are her qualifications? Look to see how many years of study she's completed, how long she's been in practice, and whether she has published any journal articles, case studies, or other writings. Publications can help your assessment in two ways: 1) you might be able to read them for yourself to get a feel for her perspective and expertise, and 2) if her work appeared in a peer-reviewed journal, it means she produced an original contribution to the field that met professional standards and is a sign of a certain degree of competence.
- What are her areas of specialty, if any? Does she have clinical experience working with clients who have similar symptoms and goals to yours? If not, she could still be a good fit as long as she's working with a mentor or supervisor who *does* have relevant experience.
- If your investigation into the first two questions has inspired your trust, the next step is to arrange to speak with the herbalist for an initial appointment or to ask a few questions. Pay attention to how you feel during and after the conversation. Feelings of distrust or discomfort are good indications that a practitioner isn't a good fit.

Other good questions to ask include:

- How long do you estimate it will take for me to see results from herbal treatment?

- What is your approach to dietary and lifestyle factors that might affect my progress?
- Do you have relationships with any medical doctors, psychotherapists, or other health professionals in the area? Who do you refer to when herbal treatment is insufficient on its own?

Look for a practitioner who has good connections with other health professionals and can give you an outline for what to expect from herbal therapies. This outline won't be a set-in-stone prediction, but it should be more specific than "everyone is different."

Recommended Suppliers

I'm happy to share some of my favorite suppliers with you. These are companies that I trust and have purchased from for years and I'm sharing them in the hopes that this list will be helpful if you're just starting out. I have no financial relationship with any company that sells herbs, supplements, or natural products, and I do not personally benefit from these recommendations in any way. Once you feel confident that you know what you're looking for, I encourage you to look for local herbalists, wildcrafters, natural food stores, and suppliers for your bulk herbs, oils, and ingredients.

Suppliers List

Bulk Herbs
- Frontier Co-op: www.frontiercoop.com
- Mountain Rose Herbs: www.mountainroseherbs.com
- Starwest Botanicals: www.starwest-botanicals.com

Tinctures and Encapsulations
- Five Flavors Herbs: www.fiveflavorsherbs.com
- Fungi Perfecti: www.fungi.com
- Gaia Herbs: www.gaiaherbs.com
- Herb Pharm: www.herb-pharm.com
- Herbalist & Alchemist: www.herbalist-alchemist.com

Essential Oils, Carrier Oils, and Body Care
- Appalachian Valley Natural Products: www.av-at.com
- Mountain Rose Herbs: www.mountainroseherbs.com
- Snow Lotus: www.snowlotus.org

Let's Stay Connected

By this point, you've gotten to know me a little bit as a teacher and a guide. If you enjoyed the way I've shared the information in this book and want to stay connected to my writing and public teaching, I'd be honored! As of the time of publication, I am an actively practicing herbalist and I work with clients from all over the United States. You can learn more about my practice, stay abreast of my teaching schedule and future publications, access free resources, and even schedule an initial consultation via my website, www.psycheandsoma.com. For free video classes and additional resources, visit my *YouTube* channel, www.youtube.com/user/MelanieStOurs.

Appendix A

RECOMMENDED READING

We herbalists joke among ourselves that this is a profession that takes multiple lifetimes to master. There's always more to learn. Growing herbs in your own garden, studying human anatomy and physiology, making new herbal recipes, and deepening your knowledge of the medicinal properties of plants are all aspects of the broader field of herbalism. Follow your interest to study the areas that appeal to you most.

Growing Medicinal Herbs

The Aromatherapy Garden: Growing Fragrant Plants for Happiness and Well-Being by Kathi Keville

Homegrown Herbs: A Complete Guide to Growing, Using, and Enjoying More Than 100 Herbs by Tammi Hartung

The Medicinal Herb Grower: A Guide for Cultivating Plants That Heal, Volume 1 by Richo Cech

Aromatherapy and Essential Oils

Aromatherapy: A Complete Guide to the Healing Art by Kathi Keville and Mindy Green

The Encyclopedia of Essential Oils: The Complete Guide to the Use of Aromatic Oils in Aromatherapy, Herbalism, Health, and Well-Being by Julia Lawless

The Healing Intelligence of Essential Oils: The Science of Advanced Aromatherapy by Kurt Schnaubelt, PhD

Making Herbal Remedies

Alchemy of Herbs: Transform Everyday Ingredients Into Foods and Remedies That Heal by Rosalee de la Forêt

The Herbal Medicine-Maker's Handbook: A Home Manual by James Green

The Modern Herbal Dispensatory: A Medicine-Making Guide by Thomas Easley and Steven Horne

Rosemary Gladstar's Herbal Recipes for Vibrant Health: 175 Teas, Tonics, Oils, Salves, Tinctures, and Other Natural Remedies for the Entire Family by Rosemary Gladstar

Healing with Food

Food and Healing: How What You Eat Determines Your Health, Your Well-Being, and the Quality of Your Life by Annemarie Colbin

Healing with Whole Foods: Asian Traditions and Modern Nutrition by Paul Pitchford

The Hip Chick's Guide to Macrobiotics: A Philosophy for Achieving a Radiant Mind and Fabulous Body by Jessica Porter

Herbal Medicine and Materia Medica

Adaptogens: Herbs for Strength, Stamina, and Stress Relief by David Winston and Steven Maimes

The Green Pharmacy Herbal Handbook: Your Comprehensive Reference to the Best Herbs for Healing by James A. Duke, PhD

Healing with the Herbs of Life by Lesley Tierra

The Web That Has No Weaver: Understanding Chinese Medicine by Ted J. Kaptchuk

The Wild Medicine Solution: Healing with Aromatic, Bitter, and Tonic Plants by Guido Masé

Natural Women's Health

Herbal Remedies for Women: Discover Nature's Wonderful Secrets Just for Women by Amanda McQuade Crawford

The Natural Pregnancy Book, Third Edition: Your Complete Guide to a Safe, Organic Pregnancy and Childbirth with Herbs, Nutrition, and Other Holistic Choices by Aviva Jill Romm

Taking Charge of Your Fertility: The Definitive Guide to Natural Birth Control, Pregnancy Achievement, and Reproductive Health by Toni Weschler

Appendix B

US/METRIC CONVERSION CHART

VOLUME CONVERSIONS	
US Volume Measure	Metric Equivalent
⅛ teaspoon	0.5 milliliter
¼ teaspoon	1 milliliter
½ teaspoon	2 milliliters
1 teaspoon	5 milliliters
½ tablespoon	7 milliliters
1 tablespoon (3 teaspoons)	15 milliliters
2 tablespoons (1 fluid ounce)	30 milliliters
¼ cup (4 tablespoons)	60 milliliters
⅓ cup	90 milliliters
½ cup (4 fluid ounces)	125 milliliters
⅔ cup	160 milliliters
¾ cup (6 fluid ounces)	180 milliliters
1 cup (16 tablespoons)	250 milliliters
1 pint (2 cups)	500 milliliters
1 quart (4 cups)	1 liter (about)

WEIGHT CONVERSIONS	
US Weight Measure	Metric Equivalent
½ ounce	15 grams
1 ounce	30 grams
2 ounces	60 grams
3 ounces	85 grams
¼ pound (4 ounces)	115 grams
½ pound (8 ounces)	225 grams
¾ pound (12 ounces)	340 grams
1 pound (16 ounces)	454 grams

INDEX

ABOUT THE AUTHOR

MELANIE ST. OURS is a clinical herbalist specializing in women's health and mental health. She is the founder of Psyche & Soma LLC, the home of her private herbal practice since 2012. For more information and free resources, visit PsycheandSoma.com.